Blaine, Tom R
Prevent that heart attack!

Date Due

MAR 1 6 1982	MAY 9 1990	JUN 2 8 1994	DEC 6
MAR 2 4 1983	MAR 8 1991	1 7 1990	DEC 2 0 2002
SEP 6 1983	APR 1 8 1992	SEP 1 9 1996	
DEC 1 0 1983	MAY 3 1993	NOV 1 2 1996	
NOV 2 6 1984	JUL 2 1990	APR 2 6 1997	
AUG 2 8 1985	NOV 9 1990		
APR 2 5 / DEC 7	NOV 23, 1991	MAY 2 1997	
	DEC 2 7	OCT 2 7 1997	
FEB 9 1989		AUG 2 4 1998	
OCT 2 7 1989	APR 1 0 1992	OCT 1 4 1999	
DEC 2 1989	FEB 0 8 1994	NOV 21 2002	

PREVENT THAT HEART ATTACK!

By the same author

GOODBYE ALLERGIES

MENTAL HEALTH THROUGH NUTRITION

CONTENTS

To Kent Blaine, my son.

FIRST EDITION

Published by Citadel Press, Inc., a subsidiary of Lyle Stuart, Inc., 120 Enterprise Avenue, Secaucus, N.J. 07094. Published ismultaneously in Canada by George J. McLeod, Limited, 73 Bathurst Street, Toronto 2B, Canada. Manufactured in the United States of America. Library of Congress Catalog Card Number 72-85522. Designed by Joan Mudgett.

ISBN 0-8065-0299-1

JUDGE TOM R. BLAINE

PREVENT THAT HEART ATTACK!

Introduction by Dr. Evan V. Shute, F.R.C.S.

THE CITADEL PRESS SECAUCUS, NEW JERSEY

INTRODUCTION

IT IS AS REFRESHING as novel to see a judge write a book on nutrition. But it reinforces the observation that war is too important to be left to generals and nutrition too vital to be left to the medical profession.

After all, the public has been conducting a controlled study on nutrition for centuries, in various geographic areas, using foods varying with latitude and custom, with occasional brilliant experiments by such ordinary folk as Sir Walter Raleigh, Jaques Cartier, or Captain Cook. Nearly every variable has been well controlled, if only by time and circumstances—if we could and would read the evidence. Unfortunately, the mass of data has been neglected, even when urged on us by a Dr. Lind. It still is in most medical schools. Nutrition is generally infra dig to doctors—not of comparable value to anatomy or pharmacology or obstetrics. Yet everyone is vitally involved, willy-nilly. And nutrition borders so closely on biochemistry that it becomes a science in spite of our neglect.

Judges and sailors and lumberjacks should discuss nutrition. Why not? It's their common bond.

There are two things we should emphasize, first about vitamin E and second about cholesterol.

Vitamin E deserves a trial in cardiovascular conditions because it has been advised for these by hundreds of investigators in the last twenty-seven years. That is a lot of experience, and hundreds of workers don't corroborate a mindless mistake. Alternative treatments are so ineffective and patients demanding treatment are so numerous that there is no good reason why this suggestion should be further ignored. Cardiovascular disease is not the atom bomb that ticks; this is the one that has exploded and killed its millions already. To see is to believe—but first I suggest that everyone should look.

Cholesterol has been widely and wildly indicated as the villain on the arteriosclerotic stage. Does everyone still hiss it? No! Just read Pinckney's recent review (E. R. Pinckney, *Medical Counterpoint*, May 1971, p. 37), then come to your own conclusion as to this villainous substance. Then recall that there are African tribes like the Masai or Samburu or Rendelle, or people like our own North American Eskimos, all of whom seem to thrive on cholesterol, and seem to dodge the cardiovascular disease that so regularly bowls us over. Do you still believe that cholesterol is the villain? I don't. Cholesterol is not a word for medical science, but an ensign of medical bankruptcy. I prefer the Rokstansky-Duguid theory.

So, good luck to another book on nutrition. Enough of these and the public will be roused to better eating and I hope to better health. Judge food as well as felons, your Honour, and serve truth at table as well as in the statutes.

Evan V. Shute, F.R.C.S. (C)

February 1972

PREFACE

HOW WOULD YOU like to enter a hospital for major surgery where the staff surgeons knew no more about surgery than was known by physicians in 1872? "Preposterous," you say, but how much progress has medical science made in the last one hundred years in preventing the killer diseases of this age—coronary thrombosis, cancer, and diabetes? Any physician will tell you that these diseases and dozens more that fill our hospitals and make physical wrecks of those who survive are increasing every year at a rate far in excess of the population increase.

It is true that doctors are more skilled than ever before in treating diseases. New drugs are available to speed recoveries and save lives.

Unfortunately, in the field of mental health the record made in recent years in preventing and treating illness has been terrible. Fabulous amounts of money, both public and private, have been available for research to psychiatrists who stubbornly cling to Freudian theories as to the causes of mental illness. In one way modern-day psychiatrists have excelled all other members of the medical profession, and that is in their suicide rate, which is four times the suicide rate of the general white population.

A world of medical proof has been accumulated that cancer is a disease caused by vitamin and mineral deficiencies. What has been the reaction of most physicians to these recent nutritional discoveries? They have responded as they always do to anything that does not correspond with the orthodox or conventional theories of the medical profession—with scorn, contempt, and ridicule.

If a thousand reputable physicians come forward with convincing proof that cancer or any other major illness can be prevented by nutrition, organized medicine will inform the public "there is no scientific evidence to substantiate such claims."

The stock answers of physicians to anything new in nutrition as a means of attaining or keeping physical and mental health are:

1. Issuance of false and untrue statements concerning possible dangers from taking harmless vitamins. Every available news media is continually used to frighten people about the dangers of taking vitamins without doctors' prescriptions. These "scare stories" come from physicians who admit in their medical journals that they know little about nutrition and that it is not taught in medical schools!

2. The old "balanced diet" myth, a figment of the imagination, which has caused millions of Americans to die or be crippled from our diseases of civilization, is dragged out and paraded for all to read and hear. Any intelligent layman knows that when important and necessary vitamins and minerals are processed out of our foods by the milling and other manufacturing industries, we are not going to get the nutrients necessary for health regardless of how much food we eat.

Physicians who vehemently assert that "a balanced

diet" gives us all of the vitamins and minerals our bodies require are nineteenth-century doctors who should move forward in their profession at least seventy years.

At the turn of the century, Americans ate a balanced diet because their foods contained the vitamins and minerals necessary for good health. Cardiovascular diseases, cancer, and diabetes were practically unknown in our great grandparents' time.

No amount of misrepresentation about vitamins changes the fact that they are foods and not drugs. Courageous researchers have shown us how we can avoid heart attacks, strokes, and a host of other diseases by following a sensible nutritional program and observing other well-known rules of health.

Not all physicians are indifferent about helping us retain good health. Conscientious doctors are fully aware that preventive medicine is in its early infancy in the United States. Will our future physicians be concerned only in treating illnesses with drugs, and in surgery, or will they be doctors for the healthy as well as the diseased?

Tom R. Blaine

PREVENT THAT HEART ATTACK!

1 A NATION OF INVALIDS

DR. PAUL DUDLEY WHITE, famed heart specialist, recently said: "When I graduated from medical school in 1911, I had never heard of coronary thrombosis, which is one of the chief threats to life in the United States and Canada today—an astonishing development in one's own lifetime! There can be no doubt but that coronary heart disease has reached epidemic proportions in the United States, where it is now responsible for more than 50 per cent of all deaths. . . . The truth is, an ever-increasing number of young men are being struck down before the age of 40 (including a large number of physicians) at the time they are most needed by their families and when they are prepared to make their greatest contribution to society."

We are told by physicians that half of all American men over forty are statistically scheduled for heart attacks. The death certificates of a majority of adults show that they died from some kind of circulatory disease.

According to Dr. William B. Kannel of Framington Heart Study, Massachusetts, one out of every four Americans is a candidate for heart attack. The person who is prone to have a fatal heart attack is described as sedentary, flabby, middle-aged, smokes cigarettes excessively, and has a diet rich in saturated fats and sugar. He will have high blood pressure and a rapid pulse at rest.

Cholesterol and stress are blamed by doctors for our failing hearts and the crippling strokes that make invalids of hundreds of thousands every year.

Our people sixty years ago and longer did not have heart attacks and strokes. They ate all the animal fat that was available. They did not trim the fat from the meat and the principal diet of many of our ancestors was pork fat, butter, cheese, cream, and foods fried in lard or other saturated fat. They often ate a half dozen eggs at a meal.

We who live today have no conception of what stress is when we consider what the pioneers went through merely to survive. Travel by foot, on horseback, or in a stagecoach—with fear of robbers and hostile Indians or wild animals—was the only way of getting from one place to another. Many of our forefathers died from starvation and cold. There was no job security for our great grandparents, and if a bank was robbed their savings, if any, were usually lost.

It is undisputed that about the time Dr. White graduated from medical school the milling industry had then adopted the process of completely stripping away the vitamins in wheat in manufacturing flour. We should remember that we eat as much sugar in two weeks as our forefathers consumed in a year.

Dr. Henry A. Schroeder of the medical school of Dartmouth University testified before a Senate subcommittee in 1970. White flour, white rice, and white sugar have lost their essential nutrients as a result of refining, said Dr. Schroeder, and are only "empty calories."

"The milling of wheat into refined white flour

removes 40 per cent of the chromium, 86 per cent of the manganese, 76 per cent of the iron, 89 per cent of the cobalt, 68 per cent of the copper, 78 per cent of the zinc, and 48 per cent of the molybdenum, all trace minerals essential for life or health. The residue of the millfeeds, which is rich in trace elements, is fed to domestic animals," said Dr. Schroeder. The trace minerals lost in the manufacture of white flour were explained by Dr. Schroeder as crucial to cardiovascular health.

You know now why cardiovascular diseases take nearly a million lives in the United States annually. We are told by physicians that 90 percent of deaths from disease involve calcium deficiency. We can avoid heart attacks and strokes by better nutrition which will lead to longer and healthier lives.

Diabetes, cancer, arthritis, and a host of other crippling diseases that are making invalids out of millions of us are largely caused by failure to get the vitamins and minerals in our foods which our ancestors ate.

Some years back one of Oklahoma's state mental hospitals ran out of money to feed its patients. The hospital had a large supply of peanut butter, and for a time the patients were fed peanut butter and dairy products from the hospital farm. Never before in the history of the hospital had there been such a recovery rate of the mentally ill! I related this story to a well-known west coast psychiatrist who said: "If the state had fed those patients beefsteaks, vegetables and fruits, instead of the cheap, empty calorie carbohydrates, and had given them vitamin and mineral supplements, nearly all of them would have recovered."

Without doubt, American is the most overfed and undernourished country in the world. As long as members of the medical profession keep telling us that if we are full we have all of the vitamins and minerals we need, we will continue to be physically and mentally crippled by the degenerative diseases that fill our hospitals and nursing homes and take such a toll of life.

Perhaps we can excuse our physicians for being so prejudiced against vitamin and mineral supplements when we read in the medical journals that nutrition is not taught in medical schools.

An eastern heart specialist recently wrote me: "My receptionist, who has a weight problem, knows more about nutrition that I do. Since the medical profession largely ignores nutrition in the prevention and treatment of disease, laymen nutritionists must inform the public."

Scores of physicians have told me privately: "I take vitamins and I give them to members of my family, but I don't recommend that my patients take vitamins. The medical organizations are opposed to any kind of self-medication, including taking vitamin supplements. No doctor can afford to incur the ill will of organized medicine."

A midwestern cardiologist wrote me: "I am having wonderful success in treating my coronary patients with vitamin E, but I don't tell any of them 'the heart medicine' I have prescribed is vitamin E."

When I pick up a national magazine and see a full-page advertisement against high blood pressure which recites: "Your doctor has drugs that will reduce your blood pressure," I get angry because the advertisement does not read: "There are foods and vitamin supplements which will cause your blood pressure to be normal." The last statement is just as true as the one appearing in the advertisement.

After the publication of *Goodbye Allergies*, my book on hypoglycemia, or low blood sugar, I received thousands of letters from readers. Ninety-nine percent of those who wrote me asked for the name and address of a physician who could cure them of hypoglycemia. That is the trouble with most of us; after we become ill we want to go right on living the way we have always lived and we hope to find a doctor who will give us some magic pill that will make us well.

The Lancet, on September 10, 1966, gave this picture of the average British citizen: "We are rapidly becoming a nation of medicine drinkers . . . we can't sleep without a sleep-maker, digest without a digestive, face the day without a stimulative, sedative, or both together, relieve Nature without a Nature-reliever." How accurately this describes, in general, a "*well*" American!

If you follow the nutritional recommendations of this book, take a reasonable amount of exercise daily, and do not attempt to commit suicide with drinking and smoking, how long should you live? I should think you can have reasonably good health, physical and mental, barring accidents, until you are 90 or 100 years old.

Biologists tell us the life span of a species is from seven to fourteen times the period one of the species takes to reach maturity. Humans mature at 20 to 25 years of age, so our life expectancy should be considerably more than 100 years.

Dr. Edward L. Bortz, a famous Philadelphia medical consultant, in his book *Creative Aging*, said there is no reason one should not live to be 100 years old. "Maybe we will someday live out our true life span of 150 years," continued Dr. Bortz. An adequate daily intake of vitamins A, B, C, D, and E is essential to long life, according to Dr. Bortz.

Good nutrition should begin in infancy and continue throughout life. Many physicians have pointed out that the aging process begins at birth and goes on through childhood, adolescence, and adult life. The one thing Dr. Bortz stressed is that every disease has a nutritional component, and the better your nutrition is the better your body is able to prevent illness or cope with it when it strikes.

Dr. William Kaufman used vitamin injections and supplements to treat over six hundred older patients with joint immobility, lack of muscular working capacity and strength, and certain mental syndromes with remarkable success.

Dr. F. J. Stare in *Nutrition and Aging* concluded that the need for sound nutrition in the elderly is not materially different from that in younger adults.

Of course, we cannot expect to live to an advanced age merely by gulping down a few vitamin and mineral supplements each day. As Dr. Bortz told us, we must have a balanced diet; keep clean; get plenty of rest; have a sense of humor and avoid the passions of hate, anger, envy, and jealousy; not overlook companionship, recreation, and pride in our jobs; keep an open mind and participate in community affairs.

If you are over 60 years old, your doctor may have told you that you should expect to have higher blood pressure than you had when you were 30. He may have suggested that your arthritis, osteoporosis, cancer, or heart disease are conditions that are a normal part of the aging process. The belief of many physicians that the problems of aging are inevitable with advancing years was shown to be false by the American Medical Association Committee on Aging in a report made in August 1963. The report reads, in part: "There are no diseases resulting from the passage of a certain number of years. . . . Neither disease nor deterioration in later years is inevitable, but there is promise of preventing, or at least postponing, such deterioration through modifying the individual's human environment. . . . All that we call the 'problems of aging'–the shaky hand, the wobbly step, the narrowing of physical and mental horizons–are not just the inevitable result of being old in years."

Recently, I was a guest at a civic club luncheon where the speaker was a young physician who talked on how one should take care of himself following a heart attack. He was asked by members of the club if there were any particular foods to avoid and if sugar and salt should be used sparingly. He answered: "I can see that some of you have been listening to the food faddists. I only limit my heart patients to a reduction in saturated fats." I had an intense desire to shout: "Don't you read the medical journals?" Since I was a guest I kept still. After the meeting, I asked the doctor if he would like me to send him copies of dozens of articles I had clipped from medical journals showing that sugar and salt might be lethal to one who had a bad heart. His answer was "no." He said he didn't have time to read his own medical magazines.

In this book I shall attempt to show how cardiovascular diseases can be prevented by nutrition, exercise, and good living habits. If you should have a heart attack or a stroke, you will need the services of a physician just as quickly as it is possible to get one and you must be hospitalized immediately. Your only hope of recovery is to follow your doctor's instructions completely and take any and all medication prescribed.

In short, I am writing for the layman who is not crippled as a result of some circulatory disease. I shall not attempt to usurp the duties of the physician who is trained to treat diseases with drugs or medication. All of the vitamin and mineral supplements I recommend that you take can be purchased "over the counter" without prescriptions. I have made a study of every medical article available on what vitamins are harmless and what vitamins can be harmful and all of this will be fully explained to you.

We have heard a lot about "minimum daily requirements" of vitamins and minerals. I hope you will think of the M.D.R. of vitamins as I do–the M.D.R. of vitamin C is enough to keep one from having scurvy; the M.D.R. of vitamin D is sufficient to prevent rickets; and so forth. As Dr. Roger J. Williams, Professor of Biochemistry at the University of Texas, said in his book, *You Are Extraordinary*, we can't solve nutritional problems on an "average individual" basis. Dr. Williams showed how people respond differently to several common drugs. In his testimony before the Federal Food and Drug Administration, opposing the proposed ban on the purchase of vitamin supplements by laymen without doctors' prescriptions, Dr. Williams said: "They cannot deny the validity of the principle of *insurance*. We do not buy fire insurance because we *know* we are going to have a fire. We do not fasten our seat belt because we *know* that our car or plane in which we ride is going to be involved in an accident. . . . There surely must be room in our country for the legitimate sale of nutritional insurance in the form of food supplements. The use of such supplements need not rest on *knowing* that we are deficient. The facts of individuality suggest strongly that deficiencies are widespread and that nutritional insurance makes sense."

As a researcher, Dr. Williams has shown that some rats live and thrive on foods when other rats die on the same foods. His conclusion is that each of us is different—a vitamin requirement for one person may be wholly inadequate for another person.

2 CHOLESTEROL AND STRESS MYTHS

WE HAVE ALL READ the scare stories about cholesterol and how it causes heart attacks. Cardiologists have been urging the public to eat less saturated animal fats and consume more polyunsaturated fats to reduce cholesterol levels. We have been taught that cholesterol is our number one enemy.

One thing we have not been told is that we cannot live without cholesterol. The uses of cholesterol in the body are so numerous that it would make this chapter too long merely to enumerate them. Those who have educated us to fear cholesterol have failed to tell us that the body makes its own cholesterol even when we eat no fats.

The anticholesterol people have conveniently overlooked telling us that the foods highest in cholesterol content are the richest in necessary nutritional ingredients—liver, kidneys, and eggs. Many people have been led to erroneously believe that, if they eat a few teaspoons of unsaturated fat every day, they need have no fear of coronary trouble.

The highly respected New York nutritionist, Dr. Norman Jolliffe, best known for his famous *Prudent Diet*, demonstrated that heart attacks can be reduced by a sensible diet with reduced consumption of fats. One of the best statements debunking the idea that cholesterol always means trouble is from the noted Canadian nutritionist, the late Dr. W. J. McCormick:

"It is quite true that a high level of cholesterol in the blood is associated with heart disease; it seems quite possible that this condition may be caused by an inability to assimilate this substance in the body rather than by too much of it in one's food." Other physicians have shown that, while too much cholesterol may be dangerous, too little cholesterol in the body would present more serious problems.

Responding to the urging by well-known physicians and the American Heart Association, untold millions of Americans have, within the past ten years, eliminated saturated fats from their diets. The heart attack rate has not been lowered, but has risen by "leaps and bounds" each year.

Harold A. Kahn of the National Heart and Lung Institute in Bethesda, Maryland, made a comprehensive report in the July 1970 issue of the *American Journal of Clinical Nutrition* on diet in the United States from 1909 to 1965. He showed that while deaths from coronary thrombosis had gone from zero to about a million a year, cholesterol levels did not increase during that half-century period of time.

As early as December 1961, *Today's Health*, an official publication of the American Medical Association, reported: "The weight of medical evidence now suggests that the amount of cholesterol in human tissues is not directly related to the amount in the diet. Since the body makes its own cholesterol, the total tissue cholesterol is about the same regardless of the amount consumed."

A fifteen-year study by the Hungarian Academy of Sciences published in 1965 in Budapest suggested that protecting against the formation of plaques of solid matter in the arteries is done by elements in the diet—specifically, vitamins A and E.

Another article in *Nutrition Reviews* (May 1969) presented evidence that the levels of heart-endangering cholesterol and triglycerides in the blood may have a strong relationship to whether or not there is enough vitamin A in the liver.

Dr. Weitzel, a German research scientist, reported in 1952 that cholesterol-fed animals developed deposits of cholesterol in the arteries while those given vitamins A and E did not have such deposits after cholesterol feedings.

In a report from the Inter-Society Commission for Heart Disease Resources, released in December 1970, more than 150 cardiovascular specialists and representatives of 29 leading health organizations admitted that as yet there is no final proof that fats and cholesterol *cause* heart disease in man.

Within the past year or so hundreds of thousands have been frightened into going to doctors to have their cholesterol and triglyceride serum levels tested. When tests showed the serum levels were above normal, the physicians seldom told the worried and frightened patients that there were harmless foods, including vitamin supplements, that would lower the cholesterol and triglyceride serum levels.

Instead, doctors have truthfully said that there were a number of drugs available for that purpose and recommended the use of one or more of such drugs. One thing the physicians probably didn't know is that anticholesterol drugs may actually harm the heart instead of helping it.

While the medication is bringing the cholesterol and triglyceride levels within normal range, it has destroyed the vitamin E in the body. *So the drug that reduces the fatty substances in your bloodstream has robbed you of the single most important nutrient for heart health in your body*!

Last year I became a victim of the disease, "cholesterol-triglyceride phobia." What frightened me most were the many medical articles I read urging cholesterol and triglyceride tests where there were family histories of coronary disease. My five brothers and sisters have all been heart victims. Most of the relatives on my mother's side had heart attacks or strokes.

I went to a heart specialist and asked his advice. "With the family history you have you should not only be tested for cholesterol and triglyceride, but you should have all of the available tests for possible cardiovascular trouble," he said. Two days later I returned to his office eager to know, but fearful of what he had found.

"I have good news for you," he reported. "Cholesterol and triglyceride are below normal. Your heart is in excellent condition; your blood pressure is low normal; there is only a trace of hardening of the arteries; in fact, your arteries are soft and pliable, and your heartbeat, after exertion, is not high. I have never before examined a 76-year-old man who had such a youthful cardiovascular system."

Then I said the wrong thing. I remarked: "Doctor,

I think the vitamin and mineral supplements I take are responsible for what your tests show." He angrily snapped back: "The vitamins and minerals had nothing to do with it. You have been wasting your money. It is all a matter of heredity."

Dr. Wilfrid E. Shute, famous cardiologist and author of *Vitamin E for Ailing and Healthy Hearts*, without doubt, has successfully treated more heart patients than any other physician in the western hemisphere. He has gained world-wide recognition for his experiences with thousands of cardiovascular patients and vitamin E.

Dr. Evan V. Shute, his brother and Medical Director of The Shute Institute, was asked at a medical meeting in Chicago on December 6, 1970, about reducing high cholesterol. His answer was: "In the first place, I don't care about high cholesterol. I think that is a 'red herring.' In the second place, I don't think that vitamin E has much influence on cholesterol levels, and I don't care. I haven't done my own cholesterol for 25 years, and I don't intend ever to do it. I don't care what it is." Again he was asked: "Does vitamin E help control cholesterol?" His answer was: "I don't know or care." Dr. Shute was quick to remind some doctor who had referred to vitamin E as a drug that vitamin E and other vitamins are *foods*.

My study of all the available books and medical articles on high cholesterol and nutrients indicates that vitamins prevent the formation of plaques of solid matter on the walls of the arteries. These plaques narrow the available space for the passage of blood and can shut off an artery. Sometimes these plaques break away from the blood vessels and close a narrow point of flow into the heart.

Our ancestors went through life with high levels of blood cholesterol, but did not have heart attacks because they ate foods rich in vitamins and minerals which prevented the formation of the deadly plaques in the bloodstream which now kill or cripple millions each year.

While most medical men and women scoff at nutrition as a preventive of heart disease, they are quick to accept and use an unproven drug in an attempt to lower cholesterol readings. Medical articles show these adverse side effects from prescribed drugs to lower cholesterol: nausea, vomiting, skin rashes, loss of hair, drawing of the skin, and kidney troubles.

The most reckless attempt to lower cholesterol has been by surgery. That part of the small intestine where dietary cholesterol is normally absorbed into the blood has been removed by surgeons. According to *Nutrition Reviews* (January 1967), the results of this type of surgery have been "particularly disappointing." Not only have patients failed to show any improvement, but death rates have been high following surgery to correct high cholesterol levels.

Dr. Wilfrid E. Shute recently wrote: "By now, most cardiologists must know they have nothing to offer but diagnosis and vague theories of the causation of a plague which threatens to engulf us as no plague or world war has ever been able to do. Many of these must know that there is a proven answer to the problems of clots. Certainly all surgeons must know of

Dr. Alton Ochsner's work. How can it possibly be ignored longer?"

Dr. Shute further said: "My father saw few cases of coronary occlusion and few diabetics. I have seen thousands. There was no coronary thrombosis in 1900. There need be none in the year 1980. . . . I think that what is good enough for the astronauts is good enough for the American citizen, who pays for their training and the many thousands of workmen and scientists who are involved in each flight. If they can get vitamin E, why can't everyone?"

Tom and Alice Fleming in *Cosmopolitan* for June 1962 defined stress as too much of anything. Stress can mean too much work, too much play, even too much exercise. Too much sunlight that causes the skin to age is an example of stress.

No one will disagree with the view that an ill person, regardless of the kind of illness, should avoid stress. We have all read the stories about the ambitious, energetic, driving business executive being a prime candidate for heart disease. We have been lulled into the false belief that all we have to do is "slow down" and avoid saturated fats to be assured of not having coronary thrombosis.

A few years ago I suddenly discovered that my heartbeat was slightly irregular. I hurried to a heart specialist who, after listening to my heartbeat, told me that I should have a complete examination, including X-ray and electrocardiogram. After all tests were completed, the physician said: "We do not find anything wrong with your heart. What you have is in the nature of a premature heartbeat. It is a fairly common occurrence and nothing dangerous. It is caused by hypertension and stress."

"But, doctor," I remonstrated, "how can I have hypertension with blood pressure of 124 over 80? I have been on vacation for nearly a month, just loafing, so I don't see how stress could be involved." The doctor gave no indication that he heard what I said. He handed me two prescriptions. "These two medications should take care of your irregular heartbeat. I would like to see you in three weeks."

The pharmacist to whom I gave the prescriptions said: "I'll be glad to fill this prescription for 24 vitamin B complex capsules because we get twice as much for vitamins by prescription as we do for those sold over the counter. Didn't you purchase a bottle of 100 vitamin B capsules three or four days ago? As for the other prescription, I would think you are the last person in this town who needs to go on a tranquilizing drug."

After I had torn up the prescriptions, I tried to recall what I had done differently on my vacation than while working. I remembered I had drunk coffee for the first time in several years. I stopped coffee drinking and have not had an irregular heartbeat since then.

Dr. Wilfrid E. Shute in the book I have just mentioned said that stress probably has little to do with heart disease. Dr. Howard B. Sprague, Boston cardiologist and former president of the American Heart Association, stated that "one man's stress is just another man's challenge."

Look around among your friends and neighbors who

have had heart attacks and determine how many of them were hard-driving, ambitious business executives. Count up how many housewives, employees, students, even retired people you know who are on tranquilizers. I was told recently that in a certain block in a well-to-do section of our town, one or more members of every family in that block regularly took tranquilizing drugs.

It is my opinion that if the millions of my fellow citizens who can't get through the day without the prescribed tranquilizing drugs would daily experience the stress of taking exercise and enjoying some type of recreation, coronary heart disease would be lowered. I have found nothing as relaxing and sleep-provoking as tired muscles.

Jokingly, but truthfully, I have often remarked that I have taken only ten sleeping pills in my 77 years and those were in hospitals following surgery. Six of those times the nurses waked me to remind me it was time to take my sleeping pills.

Dr. Hans Selye in his book, *The Stress of Life*, stated that allergic symptoms are nothing more than the body's reaction to stress. When an allergy sufferer goes to a physician for relief, he will probably be given a dangerous drug, ACTH or cortisone. Dr. T. Ogawa in *The American Journal of Physiology* (1960) said that pantothenic acid (one of the B vitamins) is just as effective with an allergy patient as are steroid preparations.

In 1954 Iowa physicians gave volunteers from a state prison food that was adequate except for a deficiency of pantothenic acid. During the second week these men became fatigued and had difficulty staying awake. By the fourth week they were quarrelsome, discontented, and miserable. They developed low blood pressure, stomach disorders, and respiratory infections (*Proceedings of the Society of Biology, 1954*).

We know how important is pantothenic acid to the proper functioning of the adrenal glands. When we consider how much stress these Iowa volunteer prisoners were under after being deprived of only *one* member of the vitamin B family for a month, we can understand why one who goes through life with deficiencies of many vitamins and minerals is a candidate for heart attack.

Many doctors say that migraine is a form of allergy. Nearly all physicians concede that migraine is a difficult disease to cure and medical literature has offered many suggestions as to possible causes of migraine. Only one who has suffered migraine attacks knows the pain that goes with the stress of this disease.

Dr. Miles Atkinson, a New York physician, reported in *Archives of Otolaryngology* (1962) that migraine results from a deficiency of vitamin B_3, or niacin. Dr. Atkinson further stated: "Those who are subject to migraine are said to be tense, rigid, perfectionist people . . . the physician who tells his migraine patient 'to take it easy' is not giving helpful advice.

"Then comes the question, routinely asked by critics and by those to whom the conception of chronic vitamin deficiency is new or unacceptable—why the deficiency, particularly in a prosperous and well-fed country such as the United States? I have no certain knowledge as to why such deficiencies arise, but we do have a number of suggestive leads. For instance, it is common knowledge that the diet of a great many people is far from ideal—the rich eat too much fat, and the poor eat too little protein and the in-betweens eat too much carbohydrates. Some eat too much in order to comfort themselves; others eat too little in order to fashion themselves. The diet records of most of the patients I see in my office make dismal reading. But intake is only one aspect of nutrition. What about absorption?" Dr. Atkinson then went on to discuss how diseases and drugs interfere with absorption and utilization of vitamins.

Several tests have been made on commercial airplane pilots to determine the effect of tension or stress on the body vitamins of the pilots. Two important results were demonstrated:

1. Immediately before the performance of a task the pilots knew would involve nervous tension, the amount of vitamins ordinarily manufactured in the body was reduced.

2. Following stressful acts, the supply of body vitamins was lower than it was preceding the period of tension.

These tests were done with men who had adequate vitamin and mineral nutrition. They were not ready to have heart attacks at the slightest provocation. What about the man who is on an average American diet? Let's listen to what experts on the subject have to say:

"Most Americans, even though they think they eat well-balanced meals, are actually lacking in certain elements and would benefit from a good vitamin and mineral supplement." Dr. H. Curtis Woods, Jr., famous nutritionist.

" 'Empty calorie' foods fail to provide adequate protein, vitamins, and essential minerals. During the past four decades, the ratio of 'empty calorie' foods in the average diet has increased so that today 'empty calorie' foods represent *one third* of the total calories consumed. *Malnutrition* is present in all age groups and at all economic and social levels." Dr. Seymour Halper, physician in charge of the New York City Department of Health Nutrition Clinic.

"To a considerable extent the perverted food habits encountered by clinical nutritionists are the creation of the food advertisers." Dr. N. Phillip Norman, noted nutritionist.

Dr. Hans Selye subjected two groups of rats to stress. One group given potassium and magnesium lived and were no worse off for the stress. The other group died from damaged heart muscles. Dr. Selye is a famous Canadian endocrinologist and medical researcher.

It is readily seen that it is not so much stress that is responsible for the ever increasing cardiovascular deaths as it is poor nutrition. Stress is one of the symptoms of a disease, *malnutrition*, that must be controlled if we are to be successful in attacking the killer diseases of this age.

3 VITAMIN E AND THE HEART

ALTHOUGH VITAMIN E was discovered about fifty years ago and has long been accepted as important in animal nutrition, it was 1959 when the United States Food and Drug Administration finally conceded that it was a necessary element in human nutrition.

Scientists estimate that in the average balanced diet some physicians are always talking about, one gets about five to seven units of vitamin E daily, perhaps less if one considers losses in cooking. These scientists believe that at the turn of the century when the United States was primarily an agricultural country, and our great-grandparents ate whatever natural foods came to them, the daily intake of vitamin E was at least 150 units per day for each person.

Researchers are demonstrating beyond doubt that this is indeed the "miracle vitamin." American physicians are dragging their feet when it comes to using this harmless and inexpensive food. This, however, can be expected. It was seventeen years after penicillin was discovered before doctors accepted it. It was about the same length of time after Dr. Samuel Levine of Boston, a great cardiologist, found that getting his heart patients out of bed as soon as they were able to sit up greatly accelerated their recovery before other physicians abandoned the practice of long bed rest in all heart cases.

We have known for some time that massive amounts of vitamin E increased the speed and endurance of racehorses. We have the testimony of countless athletes and their coaches that stamina and energy resulted from vitamin E.

We are told by newspaper and magazine stories, by radio and television interviews, and by paid advertisements in all news media, that we must eat more polyunsaturated fat to avoid heart trouble. Dr. Max K. Horwitt of the University of Illinois put men on a diet high in polyunsaturated fats, but low in vitamin E. What happened certainly wasn't what the "polyunsaturated fat" doctors anticipated. First, there was increased fragility of the red blood cells, then rupture of the blood cells which carry vital oxygen to the blood tissues. The more polyunsaturated fat the men took, the greater were the symptoms, Dr. Horwitt found.

But that wasn't all! Dr. Horwitt found that a large percentage of the men in this study developed peptic ulcers. He attributed this to the irritating effects of the rise of oxidized fat. Here we have irrefutable proof of the danger of eating polyunsaturated fats without at the same time taking adequate amounts of vitamin E.

Again, in a report to the American Chemical Society, Dr. Nicholas R. Di Luzio of Tulane University medical school found that 78 out of 81 people with a high intake of polyunsaturates developed toxic, highly oxidized fats in their blood. When he added vitamin E to the diet, even with polyunsaturated fats, the blood level of these people became normal. When he removed vitamin E from the diet, the same toxic, highly oxidized fat situation again developed.

Dr. Edward R. Pinckney, famous California internist, wrote in the May 1970 *Medical World News*, "Reports indicate that heated polyunsaturated fats and oils not only defeat the purpose allegedly intended, but are also toxic and might even be carcinogenic." Webster defines "carcinogenic" as relating to a substance or agent producing or inciting cancer.

Dr. L. M. Hursh of the University of Illinois, after warning that heated unsaturated fats strip the body of its vitamin E stores, recently said: "There is one other problem no one ever discusses and that is the co-carcinogenic activity of heated unsaturated fat. . . . This is a very serious problem, but has gained little attention."

Nutrition Reviews (September 1957) reported on the changes in animals when fed heated polyunsaturated fats as compared to heated butter. The animals fed heated unsaturated corn oil developed diarrhea, rough fur, decreased food intake, and had lower growth rates, while the butter-fed animals showed no such changes.

F. A. Kummerow in "*A Symposium on Foods*" (Oregon State University, 1961) pointed out the carcinogenic activity of heated polyunsaturates. All ninety-six animals fed heated corn oil developed tumors and only one survived a forty-month experimental period. All of the animals fed unheated corn oil survived and none of them, according to Kummerow, had cancerous growths.

Drs. M. L. Pierce and S. Dayton (*Journal of the American Medical Association*, December 28, 1970) reported to the American Heart Association that men on experimentally high polyunsaturated fat diets had

65 percent greater incidence of cancer than did a control group given a standard diet. Drs. Pierce and Dayton said that their unexpected finding "raised a red flag" on proposals to substitute vegetable oil fats for animal fats for the entire population.

Dr. George Mann, Professor of Biochemistry at Vanderbilt University (*Medical World News*, August 28, 1970) characterized the fatty acid diet approach to coronary heart disease as a "myth." He said that physicians who had tried the diet therapy for hypercholesteremia and heart disease had found that "it doesn't work."

It should be observed that Germany has banned the reuse by reheating of polyunsaturated fats in commercial cooking.

Other tests have shown that polyunsaturated fats burn faster than saturated fats, so the body needs a greater amount of vitamin E to maintain proper control of metabolism. This does not mean we should never eat polyunsaturated fats; however, unless we provide the body with more oxygen which can only come from vitamin E, we are in trouble on a polyunsaturated fat diet.

Dr. Aloys Tappel, famed University of California nutritionist, at a 1970 meeting of the Federation of American Societies for Experimental Biology, reported that destruction of fat by oxygen is the basic cause of the aging cell. Dr. Tappel called this a "universal disease" which could be slowed by increased use of antioxidants. He pointed out that abnormal oxidation of fats in a cell is almost completely suppressed by vitamin E.

In 1969, after many medical reports showed that infants fed formulas containing polyunsaturated fats developed irritability, swelling, skin lesions, and changes in red blood cells, the American Academy of Pediatrics recommended that vitamin E be used in all infant formulas.

Most of the medical literature on vitamin E relates to the dramatic recoveries of heart patients who have been given this vitamin in massive amounts after heart attacks. The famed Drs. Shute of the Shute Institute, London, Ontario, Canada, have treated over thirty-thousand such patients with therapies including vitamin E. Other physicians all over the world have discovered that vitamin E is a fibrinolysin, exerting its effect on the fibrin-fibrinolysin equilibrium in the bloodstream, and on the lining of the vessels. While circulating in the bloodstream vitamin E prevents dangerous thrombi from forming.

Dr. E. Cheraskin and Dr. W. M. Ringsdorf, Jr., of the University of Alabama, gave a report in the August 1970 issue of *Nutrition Report International* on Vitamin E. Four hundred and thirty-three individuals were studied—all professional people and members of their families. Eighty percent of these educated and affluent people were getting less vitamin E than was needed as a bare minimum! The report continued:

"The data confirm the well-established fact that, with advancing age, there are progressively more cardiovascular symptoms and signs."

This startling result was shown by Drs. Cheraskin

and Ringsdorf: "Cardiovascular findings do indeed increase with age, but only in those subjects consuming sub-optimal amounts of vitamin E."

A year later another dietary and cardiovascular survey was made with the same subjects. Summarizing their later findings, Drs. Cheraskin and Ringsdorf reported: "During this (one year) interval, those who increased vitamin E intake were paralleled by a decrease in cardiovascular symptoms and signs. Those who did not increase vitamin E consumption did not improve with regard to the clinical picture."

While the proof is conclusive that clots in the arteries can be dissolved with the harmless vitamin E, doctors continue to ridicule vitamins and prescribe dangerous anticoagulant drugs for clots or arterial occlusion. A report in the September 1, 1961, *Journal of the American Medical Association* by Dr. Russell L. Miller of the University of Michigan told of three cases of bleeding into the pericardium, the sac that surrounds the heart, following administration of an anticoagulant drug.

The antioxidant property of vitamin E enables the blood to carry oxygen to the tissues so that the heart requires less oxygen to do its work. Vitamin E is also a vasodilator that expands the arteries so that blood can be easily and smoothly circulated. Vitamin E's anticoagulant power is the best insurance we can have against coronary attacks and strokes.

Dr. Weitzel of West Germany in 1955 at a Vitamin E Symposium in Venice pointed out that vitamins E and A are useful for arteriosclerosis. Drs. Wilfrid and

Evan Shute have successfully used the combination of vitamins E and A since 1955 in arteriosclerosis cases.

Dr. Evan V. Shute has shown that vitamin E should not be taken with inorganic iron, a form of medication, but that it may be taken with any food containing organic iron. Inorganic iron destroys vitamin E if taken at the same time.

Dr. Wilfrid E. Shute has explained that with the hypertensive (high blood pressure) and with those with a chronic rheumatic heart vitamin E should be taken with caution. "In chronic rheumatic hearts, most people can't take more than 150 units a day–hardly any ever got above 200 units a day. . . . Some hypertensives, not many, just the rare ones, show an initial upsurge of systolic pressure when you give them vitamin E in a big dose. . . . We watch for this initial upsurge of pressure. If we get by the first week without that complication, we could almost feel safe in giving any dose henceforth. There is a good chance that the blood pressure will come down," said Dr. Shute.

Dr. Evan V. Shute has observed: "There is one other warning that I should give about vitamin E, and that is in the diabetic. When we analyzed our own cases some years ago, we found that 25 per cent of the diabetics who were on insulin had a decrease of insulin requirements of ten units or more. These decreases can occur suddenly within the first 72 hours of the initiation of treatment. We caution all diabetics on insulin who begin to take vitamin E to carry some candy in their pockets for fear they will have a prompt reaction in the first two or three days. The insulin they have needed for 25 years may suddenly become much less. We have seen people taking 70 units go off it entirely, not often, but we have seen this."

Dr. Evan V. Shute further explained that if one gets a rash or nausea from vitamin E, it will usually be an allergy and can be corrected by switching to some other form of vitamin E.

It has been suggested by physicians that one going on vitamin E to prevent heart disease should take 100 units a day for a week and have his physician determine if he can then take larger doses. Recently, Dr. Evan V. Shute said: "There are a lot of unsuspected rheumatic hearts around, and a lot of murmurs, too, whose owners don't know anything about them. These people may never get to a dose higher than 150 units a day."

Occasionally, when one starts taking vitamin E, it causes a temporary rise in blood pressure which usually does no harm.

The question is asked, "How much vitamin E should one take to keep the heart healthy?" Most people take 100 to 200 units daily, which certainly should be considered the minimum. I take 800 units of vitamin E daily. I think the average adult who wants to be on the safe side will take 400 to 600 units of vitamin E each day to avoid cardiovascular disease. This is, of course, on the assumption that he is taking other vitamin supplements.

Many individuals take much larger daily amounts of vitamin E as a prophylaxis for heart trouble—say, 1,600 to 3,200 units–with no adverse results. As Dr. Evan V. Shute said: "There is no top dose for vitamin E except for chronic rheumatic hearts and people with hypertension."

Since vitamin E is fat-soluble and slowly absorbed, it should be taken at mealtime, preferably with some fat. I take all of my vitamin E supplements at breakfast as there is no advantage in dividing the amounts taken two or three times daily. Since men are more susceptible to heart disease than women, I believe they should take more vitamin supplements than should women.

Dr. Wilfrid E. Shute has told about men who were brought to him near death with coronary thrombosis, who, after extensive treatment with massive amounts of vitamin E, have had complete physical examinations by other physicians who could detect no damage to the hearts.

Angina pectoris has been called the disease of middle-aged men although men and women of all ages have it. Generally, the hardening of the coronary artery has come on gradually so the supply of blood to the heart muscle has been slowly decreased. The lack of oxygen causes dizziness and/or chest pains.

Most doctors prescribe nitroglycerine tablets or other nitrites and decreased activity for angina patients. Most physicians believe that these drugs dilate the coronary arteries and relieve pain, but this is now being widely questioned. Perhaps nobody knows how nitrites act. It is known that nitrites do not attack the cause of the disease. Vitamin E in amounts from 300 to 600 units daily reduces the oxygen requirement of the heart muscle to where individuals with mild or moderate coronary insufficiency may not require medication.

This does not mean that an angina patient can take vitamin E and handle any kind of exertion without danger. Dr. Wilfrid E. Shute has observed that eight out of ten angina patients who take vitamin E are improved. As with any other heart condition, no angina patient should attempt to dispense with the services of his physician—neither should he try to experiment with vitamin supplements without his doctor's permission.

If I should ever suffer angina pectoris, I would insist that my doctor consider vitamin E. If he told me that he knew nothing about vitamin E, I would insist that he read Dr. K. L. Zierler's article (1948) in the *American Journal of Physiology*, wherein he said that if vitamin E is present in the bloodstream, blood clots will not occur.

I hope you will enjoy the continuation of our trip into a wonderful fairyland of nutrition where foods and not drugs help us to lead longer, healthier, and happier lives than we had ever anticipated.

4 B VITAMINS AND THE HEART

ALL VICTIMS OF heart failure have one thing in common—they are malnourished. Drs. Joseph G. Pittman and Phin Cohen—in the April 20, 1964, issue of the *New England Journal of Medicine*—warned that malnutrition is the usual aftermath of heart failure. These physicians noted that loss of appetite or lack of interest in food is common to many diseases, especially congestive heart failure.

Sometimes, because of the patient's overweight, the physician imposes dietary restrictions on foods the patient likes best. We all know that a big meal puts a strain on a bad heart. A cardiac patient with abdominal pain and swelling of the abdomen along with difficult breathing will normally find his appetite reduced.

A heart patient expends abnormal amounts of energy. A fast heartbeat, a rise in temperature, excessive sweating, and nervous system activities use more of the patient's energies than were used before the heart attack. This requires increased oxygen consumption, so vitamin E intake becomes important, in fact, essential.

The demands of the breathing muscles, the heart muscle, and the blood manufacturing system must be met in some manner. Some heart patients have fever in the early stages of the disease. These patients must have increased nutrition and since they cannot eat more they must have vitamin food supplements, including vitamin E. The B vitamins are very important in any therapeutic program because they are essential to digestion and the use of foods. Any plan that does not include good nutrition is shortsighted and not in the best interests of a heart patient.

Dr. E. Cheraskin of the University of Alabama Medical Center, writing in *The International Journal for Vitamin Research* (1967), demonstrated from tests made with a large number of subjects that those with heart complaints were the ones who consumed the most carbohydrate foods with the least amount of thiamine (vitamin B_1).

Nutrition Reviews (October 1955) reviewed the result of testings made on human cadavers by M. G. Wohl and associates. A comparison of the liver and kidney tissues of those who died from severe organic heart diseases and those who died from other causes showed much less thiamine in the heart patients' tissues than in the tissues of the others examined.

Dr. Earl E. Aldinger of Tulane University medical school put rats on a thiamine-free diet for five weeks. The animals had erratic heartbeats and the tissues surrounding the hearts lost 69 percent of their tension and elasticity. Many of the rats died during the experiment.

Dr. Tibor L. Kopjas, in an article in the November 1966 issue of the *Journal of the American Geriatric Society*, reported that after extensive testing he had found folic acid (one of the B vitamins) effective in combating arteriosclerosis. It was Dr. Kopjas' conclusion that folic acid was an effective but harmless dilator of small arteries.

Dr. Henry Schroeder of Washington University school of medicine told us in *The Journal of Chronic Diseases* (July 1955) that pyridoxine (vitamin B_6) deficiency will cause hardening of the arteries and high blood pressure. Dr. Schroeder reported that losses of this vitamin through processing and cooking may make it impossible to get enough pyridoxine during winter months. "It is entirely possible that the American adult is maintained on a marginal intake of this important coenzyme (pyridoxine) during periods of the year in which fresh vegetables and fruits are not available and processed foods and meats are widely used," he said. Since many adults eat only small amounts of fresh fruits and vegetables, it is easy to understand why so many adults, particularly men, have hardening of the arteries.

Another important use of pyridoxine is to assist the body in using unsaturated fatty acids. Dr. Schroeder stated that monkeys deficient in pyridoxine have higher cholesterol levels in their blood than do monkeys fed an adequate amount of this important vitamin.

Another B vitamin, choline, has been found effective in helping reduce high blood pressure. Heretofore, little has been known about choline. Dr. W. Stanley Hartroft of the University of Toronto, in a paper in the *American Journal of Public Health* (March 1966), reported that young rats fed a choline-deficient diet developed high blood pressure.

Eggs and liver are rich in choline. Dr. Hartroft explained that young rats and young dogs deprived of choline developed high blood pressure which could not be corrected by later adding choline to the diet. He reasoned that the damage to babies from not feeding foods containing choline is not reversible. A mother who neglects to feed her infant child egg yolk and liver (in an appropriate form) is taking a chance of rearing a son or daughter who will be a hypertensive adult.

In a *Newsweek* article for September 11, 1950, Dr. Louis B. Dotti and associates of St. Luke's Hospital, New York, told of feeding inositol (a B vitamin) and cholesterol to rabbits as compared with feeding only the same amount of cholesterol to rabbits. The rabbits fed cholesterol showed a 337 percent increase in blood cholesterol while those fed cholesterol and inositol showed an increase of only 181 percent.

The same group of researchers (Dotti et al.) reported in a 1949 paper in *Proceedings of the Society of Experimental Biology and Medicine* that a group of diabetic patients fed inositol over an eight-week period showed marked decreases in cholesterol in the blood. The well-known medical facts are that most diabetics have high cholesterol levels and that vitamins A and E keep cholesterol clots or plaques from forming on arterial walls. This should cause physicians to routinely give vitamins A and E to their diabetic patients to prevent heart attacks and strokes.

As far back as 1956 newspapers reported the favorable results obtained at the Mayo Clinic by giving niacin (a B vitamin) to those with high cholesterol blood levels. In 1957 (*Nutrition Views and News*) from Canada came reports of the successful use of niacin in lowering cholesterol in both humans and animals.

In the *Canadian Medical Association Journal* in 1957 and again in 1958, and in the *British Medical Journal* in 1958, were articles by physicians showing that it had been definitely established that niacin was a valuable anticholesterol agent. *Newsweek* on November 9, 1959, stated that niacin is "the most effective way to reduce blood cholesterol levels."

It is interesting to note that in 1961 the *Medical Journal of Australia* reported that physicians in that country had found that vitamins A and D were successfully employed tools in fighting high cholesterol levels.

Although one anticholesterol drug, MER/29, was used on over four hundred thousand patients by physicians before the government stepped in and prohibited its use as causing blindness, falling hair, skin diseases, and loss of sexual desire, physicians have shown little or no interest in recommending niacin (nicotinic acid). Dr. Williams B. Parsons, Jr., director of research at the Jackson Clinic and Foundation, Madison, Wisconsin, writing in *Medical Tribune* (November 28, 1964), suggested that if niacin could be patented, physicians might use it instead of drugs. Dr. Parsons said that drug companies, without the incentive of large profits from a new drug, aren't interested in promoting a vitamin–one that can be bought over the counter without prescription.

Some physicians have objected to using niacin

because, when first taken, some subjects have a slight flushing of the skin.

A new version of nicotinic acid, "niacinamide," was developed and is now generally available, causing no flushing of the skin.

We don't definitely know why nicotinic acid (niacin) is so effective in controlling high cholesterol levels. Many researchers believe it is the result of nicotinic acid (niacin) deficiency in the body. Many doctors refuse to believe that one can have a nicotinic acid (niacin) deficiency short of pellagra.

Although he exhibits no concern about the danger of drugs that are often more harmful than the conditions for which they are given, a doctor will become greatly concerned about possible harmful side effects if you mention a vitamin or mineral supplement. Dr. Parsons reported that in some ninety patients given nicotinic acid there developed some changes in the liver enzyme functions after long continued usage. A few others developed nausea. The abnormal liver condition, which Dr. Parsons described as minor and not sufficient to discontinue the use of the vitamin, was caused by a synthetic *aluminum* nicotinic acid instead of plain nicotinic acid.

Since niacinamide has been perfected and marketed, no adverse side effects have been reported by those who have taken it as far as I have been able to ascertain.

Articles in the medical journals state that niacin is more effective than niacinamide in lowering blood cholesterol levels, while niacinamide works better than niacin in relieving arthritic conditions.

As I explained in *Mental Health Through Nutrition,* niacin—or, as it is also called, vitamin B_3—and vitamin C have for some time been used *in massive doses* in the treatment of schizophrenia. Hundreds of psychiatrists who have prescribed niacin and vitamin C in enormous amounts for mentally ill patients have reported no adverse side effects from such vitamins. With the bitter opposition of orthodox psychiatrists to the treatment of the mentally ill by any other than conventional methods, we can be certain that if there had been any bad side effects they would have received wide publicity.

MER/29, upon which William S. Merrill Company spent nearly $2 million for advertising, selling $12 million of the drug, was hailed by Dr. Arthur Ruskin of Texas at the 1960 American Medical Association meeting as "a step forward in the simple control of blood and liver cholesterol without modification of diet or danger to the patient." It is interesting to observe that, before the sale of MER/29 was banned by the government, livers of experimental animals were found to have become enlarged from the drug; it was found dangerous for a pregnant woman to take and its use was determined to be detrimental to the adrenal glands.

When we consider that the human body was able to handle its cholesterol without drugs from primitive times until after 1910 and that twentieth-century Americans who now eat what most doctors consider the finest diets in the world are plagued with cholesterol levels so high they are considered prime suspects for heart attacks, is it not time physicians and laymen consider the possibility of building healthy bodies that can control their own cholesterol levels?

We live in an age of medical specialization. How can any heart specialist contend that the drug he prescribes for cholesterol control is successful if patients suffer damage to other organs in their bodies? Why hasn't medical science tried to find out why we were able to get along for thousands of years without heart fatalities and without expensive and sometimes dangerous drugs? I think the answer to the last question is that the prevention of coronary thrombosis and other cardiovascular diseases by good diet and exercise appears to be too simple for men and women whose training has been the treatment of diseases by drugs. One who has been taught that a drug should be used where there is disease is not going to become enthusiastic about nutrition as either a preventive or cure for disease.

My opinion is that MER/29 is now the safest of all anticholesterol drugs for one reason—it has been recalled and cannot be prescribed by physicians. When cholesterol lowering drugs damage the kidneys, the liver, the skin, the hearing, and other bodily functions, isn't it time for physicians to turn to simple and harmless vitamin supplements to control cholesterol?

What B vitamins should one take to avoid heart trouble? I take one B-complex vitamin capsule, eight Brewer's yeast tablets, and two 100 mg. niacinamide tablets each day. I prefer to take all of my B vitamin supplements at breakfast time for two reasons: (1) they are water-soluble and should be taken with food, and (2) thiamine, or vitamin B_1, is an energy-producing vitamin. If I should take all of these B vitamins just before retiring, I might not be able to sleep as well as if I had taken them earlier in the day. We usually need extra energy from thiamine, or vitamin B_1, early in the day. When I know that I am going to have to stay up until very late, I wait until the evening meal to take the B vitamins.

5 VITAMIN C AND THE HEART

WE HAVE BEEN TOLD since childhood that we are as old as our arteries. If we get enough vitamin C (ascorbic acid) in our diet, the chances are that our arteries will never grow old. Dr. Boris Sokoloff of the Southern Bio-Chemical Institute of Lakeland, Florida, had an interesting article in the December 1966 issue of *The Journal of the American Geriatrics Society*. It was based on extensive experimental evidence and corroboration from medical literature.

Dr. Sokoloff and his associates are of the opinion that atherosclerosis can be avoided by sufficient intake of vitamin C. Atherosclerosis is a lesion of large- and medium-sized arteries with deposits of yellowish plaques containing cholesterol, lipoid material, and lipophages. These physicians believe that the real cause of the clogging of the arteries is the production of serum triglycerides produced by sugars and fats. To combat triglycerides, the body synthesizes an enzyme known as lipo-protein lipase, or LPL, which comes from the walls of healthy capillaries. The capillary walls depend on vitamin C for health.

Due to the action of LPL, the triglycerides and cholesterol are broken down into free fatty acids and the blood vessels are cleared. With adequate vitamin C in the body, there is no chance for fatty plaques to cling to the artery walls, clog them, and prevent the flow of blood through the arteries. If the vitamin C supply in the body is low, the arteries will get hard and brittle. Dr. Sokoloff explained that when one grows older the body has more difficulty producing LPL to control the cholesterol and lipids in the bloodstream.

Dr. Sokoloff, reporting on his group's laboratory experiments on rats and a large number of people, showed that vitamin C is not a "miracle drug" in advanced hypercholesteremia or cardiac disease cases. It takes five or six months of intensive use of vitamin C for beneficial results to appear. From this and other reports, we must conclude that if we are to avoid atherosclerosis, the forerunner of heart disease, we must have adequate amounts of vitamin C in the diet before trouble develops. Since serum triglycerides are produced more from sugar than fats, we must drastically reduce our sugar intake as well as the amount of saturated fats we eat.

Dr. Sokoloff referred to the work of Dr. M. Higuchi, an eminent Japanese physician who found that as we grow older the vitamin C we have stored in our tissues is withdrawn from the capillaries for the use of other body glands that are dependent on vitamin C. That, of course, leaves the capillaries depleted and unable to produce the LPL necessary to battle cholesterol and the triglycerides, so we develop atherosclerosis.

If you would keep your arteries from becoming clogged with fatty plaques that cling to the artery walls, a condition that may kill or cripple you suddenly and without warning, you should take vitamin C every day of your life.

You may never find the fountain of youth, but you won't be far from it when you discover what vitamin C can do for you. If you are forty and over, don't let any doctor or layman lead you to believe that arthritis, back pains, cancer, ulcers, hardening of the arteries, and heart disease are aging diseases and inevitable. There is a mountain of evidence available that vitamin C, if started in time and taken in adequate amounts, can reverse the symptoms of aging. Vitamin C is our chief protection against the toxic materials our environment forces on us daily.

Vitamin C is indispensable to the formation of collagen, a "glue-like" substance that holds our cells in a natural healthy condition. As long as collagen performs its binding job, tissues do not deteriorate, and invading infections are successfully resisted. Inflammation of the walls of the small- and medium-sized arteries of the body is one of the results when collagen is broken down.

Dr. William J. McCormick said in *Archives of Pediatrics* (October 1954): "The degree of malignancy of an illness is determined inversely by the degree of connective tissue resistance. And this, in turn, is dependent on the adequacy of vitamin C intake."

The medical magazine *MD* (January 1957) reprinted an article by two Russian scientists showing that vitamin C is a worthwhile preventive against hardening of the arteries and impaired circulation leading to heart disease. These Soviet physicians found that vitamin C increased the rate of oxidation, stimulated the liver, and thus speeded up the breakdown of cholesterol. As a protective measure against circulatory diseases, they recommended from 500 to 1,000 milligrams of vitamin C daily.

Dr. C. J. Shafar reported in the British medical journal, *The Lancet* (July 22, 1967), that what is often taken for heart disease on the reading of an abnormal electrocardiogram tracing may be a deficiency of vitamin C.

Dr. J. C. Paterson, a noted pathologist, in a recent article in *The Canadian Medical Association Journal* concluded that vitamin C deficiency is related to coronary thrombosis. He showed that 81 percent of coronary cases in hospitals have subnormal blood plasma levels of vitamin C, whereas 55.8 percent of a similar noncoronary group in the hospitals were vitamin C subnormal.

French researchers found that young people who died in prison camps in World War II had widespread arteriosclerosis and thrombosis, a condition certainly not brought on by having eaten too much saturated fats.

Morton S. Biskind said in the *Journal of Institutional Medicine* (1951) that physicians who advise against liver, eggs, and other cholesterol-rich foods impair the nutritional status of their patients. He cited records where patients put on a high vitamin regime and then given cholesterol-rich foods had dramatic reductions in the blood cholesterol levels.

As Dr. W. J. McCormick has shown, sugar, alcohol, and tobacco rob the body of vitamin C. It has been proven by laboratory tests that one cigarette destroys the vitamin C content of an average orange. Postmortem examinations of 150 cases of heavy smokers who died of coronary thrombosis showed 97 percent were deficient in vitamin C.

Dr. McCormick held that a high level of vitamin C in our bodies was our best protection against unusual stress that might trigger a heart attack. His conclusion that circulatory problems are less a matter of too much cholesterol and more problems of not enough vitamins B and C is sound and finds support in the medical literature of many countries.

Dr. Emil Ginter told the Fifth International Convention on Dietary Lipids in October 1966 that he fed cholesterol-rich foods to laboratory guinea pigs, but added 50 milligrams of vitamin C to each feeding. He also fed the same cholesterol-rich foods to other guinea pigs without added vitamin C. The animals were sacrificed and Dr. Ginter found that those who had been given vitamin C had cholesterol levels 30 to 40 percent lower than did the others.

Dr. Richard Bing of Wayne State University found that vitamin C promotes healing after myocardial infarction, which all doctors agree is a life-threatening stage of coronary disease.

Dr. Charles G. King of Columbia University school of medicine found that vitamin C determines the rate with which cholesterol accumulates in the arteries. Using guinea pigs, Dr. King discovered that animals fed a diet without vitamin C showed an increase of 600 percent in cholesterol in their bloodstreams.

In the *Journal of the American Dietetic Association* (June 1953), Dr. Sidney G. Spector said: "Almost any stress, if sufficiently severe and prolonged, will cause a lowering of the amount of ascorbic acid in the tissues." Dr. Spector found that vitamin C had great value for those who had traumatic shock, as a wound or an injury. We call attention to the well-known fact that practically all surgeons now administer vitamin C before, at the time of, and after surgery to protect their patients against the stress of surgery.

A heart patient is particularly vulnerable to stressful situations and should be given adequate amounts of vitamin C to protect him from situations that naturally arise.

Most animals synthesize their own vitamin C and are not dependent on food for this valuable vitamin. Man does not manufacture or synthesize vitamin C and is completely dependent on foods for the vitamin. The small guinea pig is one animal that cannot synthesize vitamin C and, like man, must get this vitamin from the food it eats. So guinea pigs can and do develop vitamin C deficiencies. That makes them useful in studying the effects of a lack of vitamin C, particularly as regards the arteries and heart.

Dr. Carl F. Shaffer made extensive research on guinea pigs to determine if atherosclerosis can be induced by giving them a diet free of vitamin C. His investigation showed that the lesions and damage to the arteries of guinea pigs fed no vitamin C were "identical to human atherosclerosis." We further quote from Dr. Shaffer's article in the January 1970 issue of the *Journal of Clinical Nutrition*: "There is a basis for the presumption of deficiency in ascorbic acid (as a contributory factor) in the development of myocardial, aortic and cerebral atherosclerosis."

Dr. Shaffer was, of course, referring to humans when he made the last quoted statement. He reported the atherosclerosis he found in vitamin C deficient guinea pigs as a fact and not as a presumption.

The suggestion that vitamin C deficiency is related to the killer diseases has produced no great interest among the heart specialists. Most of them are content to talk about heredity, too much saturated fats, too much stress, and being too obese.

The picture, however, is not as gloomy as one might think. This is still a free country and we can protect ourselves against heart attacks and strokes by taking lots of exercise and eating the foods we know are high in the vitamins and minerals that prevent cardiovascular diseases. At a very nominal cost we can buy the vitamin and mineral supplements our bodies require. We can drastically cut down on our sugar intake. (I'll have more to say about that later.)

How much vitamin C should one take and can one "overdose" on vitamin C? The only documented claim made against taking too much vitamin C is that with some people massive amounts of vitamin C have a slightly laxative effect. If this should occur, a reduction should be made in the amount of the vitamin taken. I take 2,000 milligrams of vitamin C daily, dividing it fairly equally with the three meals. It should be taken with other foods as it is water-soluble. I either chew up vitamin C tablets or dissolve them in fruit juice before taking since some nutritionists believe the tablets can pass through the stomach without being dissolved.

6 FOODS THAT HELP THE HEART

OUR GRANDPARENTS KNEW that "an apple a day keeps the doctor away." They believed that apples were good for us because they helped elimination. After vitamins were discovered, it was thought that the vitamin C of apples was what made them so beneficial. Now we know that it is the pectin in apples that makes them so valuable as a health food.

Pectin is important in helping rid our bodies of toxins. Dr. Ancel Keys in 1960 cited experiments to show that pectin lowers blood cholesterol. Wells and Ershoff in 1961 demonstrated that rats fed a high cholesterol diet with a pectin supplement did not show cholesterol increases in the blood and liver. *Science* reported on November 20, 1964, that dogs with hardening of the arteries showed lower cholesterol levels after being fed a standard diet with pectin. Drs. Hans Fisher and Paul Griminger of Rutgers University announced in the April 1968 issue of *Farm Journal* that apples may be important factors in preventing heart disease. They found that pectin limits the amount of cholesterol the body can absorb. Dr. Glenn H. Joseph, writing in *Nutrition Research* (September 1955), said that pectin is a natural detoxifier. Pectin ingestion has been shown to prevent lead poisoning.

Grant Palmer and David Dixon reported in the June 1966 issue of the *American Journal of Clinical Nutrition* that sixteen men with normal cholesterol levels were tested for four weeks on a diet containing pectin along with their usual food, and that "as the daily pectin dose was increased, the corresponding cholesterol was reduced."

It is not known how pectin lowers cholesterol in the blood. Some physicians believe that pectin stops the intestine from absorbing the fatty acids so that they pass on out of the body without entering the bloodstream. This theory finds support from experiments with chickens where it was found that grated apples added to a cholesterol-rich diet worked better in lowering cholesterol blood levels than did whole apples. Dr. Ancel Keys summed it up in this sentence: "It appears probable, however, that the high consumption of fruits, including apples, by some populations, helps to explain the low blood cholesterol values in those populations."

There are so many ways apples may be eaten that we should never grow tired of them. Eat them raw or cooked, as a salad food, as part of the main meal, or as a dessert. Apple juice can be taken at meal times or between meals. Italian researchers found that apple sauce, when added to the diet, stabilized cholesterol levels.

When you eat apples, you not only get the needed pectin, but generous amounts of vitamins A, B_1, B_2, and C. Raw apples are especially good for the gums and teeth. If you eat raw apples, you should peel them to get rid of the poisons resulting from spraying. Every homemaker knows the value to her family of ripe fruits as digestive aids. If you have a stomach or duodenal ulcer, cooked apples liquified in a blender are your best food to cure the ulcer. Apple pectin tablets are sold in drugstores and health food stores and are helpful in controlling cholesterol.

Lecithin is another food that has been found useful in fighting cholesterol. It is found in natural vegetable oils, beef liver, brains, kidneys, beef heart, egg yolk, wheat germ, nuts, and seeds. Most people who are frightened at the word "cholesterol" refuse to eat many or all of these nutritious foods.

Lecithin breaks down cholesterol into small particles that move easily in the bloodstream with no harm resulting. Fats, when hydrogenated, lose lecithin, so cholesterol in hydrogenated fats is dangerous because it does not have protective lecithin. The cholesterol from fats without lecithin protection collects in clumps on the arterial walls and heart disease follows.

An article in the January 1958 *Geriatrics* reported that two tablespoonfuls of lecithin given daily to patients with high cholesterol and high blood pressure reduced the cholesterol level 41 percent in thirteen out of fifteen such patients. Dr. Lester M. Morrison, prominent Los Angeles physician, recently said, "There seems to be good evidence now that in very high concentrations lecithin can also dissolve the fatty plaques in the arteries."

Egg yolk is rich in cholesterol and also in lecithin. Those doctors who are always warning us against eating eggs because of cholesterol apparently do not know that eggs have a "built-in" protection, lecithin, which makes them safe to eat. Soybeans are an excellent source of lecithin.

Drs. Pottenger and Krohn in the *American Journal*

of Digestive Disease (April 1962) told how they put their high blood pressure patients on diets high in cholesterol and lecithin made from soybeans. "The blood cholesterol showed a marked decrease in 79 per cent of the patients who took the lecithin," the report said.

Dr. Robert Hodges of the University of Iowa fed a group of healthy volunteers a soybean "meat substitute" and observed that their cholesterol levels dropped from an average of 300 to an average of 200. Dr. Hodges explained that the usual level of cholesterol in Americans is 240 milligrams per cubic centimeter.

Why has the ability of lecithin to help in the proper metabolism of cholesterol been ignored by those who claim to be so concerned about the cholesterol problem? Why have we not been told that lecithin-rich foods, or lecithin itself, will compensate for the fat intake our bodies seem to require? The foods that will be a good defense against cholesterol accumulation are high in lecithin and unsaturated fats. The heart that can and will withstand stress when it threatens us is the well-nourished heart.

Dr. John L. Simpson of the University of California told the 1957 California Academy of General Practice of his experiments with lecithin on animals. "Lecithin apparently invaded the artery walls and depleted them of fatty plaques which were then deposited in the bloodstream. Once in the bloodstream, the fat appeared to be metabolized, or burned up," said Dr. Simpson. (See *Let's Live*, March 1958.)

Dr. William G. Delamater in *Let's Live* told of a

patient he had whose cholesterol had reached the dangerous peak of nearly 1,000. By a steady use of lecithin, Dr. Delamater was able to reduce the cholesterol level of this patient to 280 in six months.

Dr. Ronald K. Tompkins of Ohio State University medical school told the Federation of American Society for Experimental Biology in April 1968 that human gallstones are composed of 90 percent cholesterol and that when lecithin is taken the chances for having "hard stones" are greatly reduced.

Lecithin's ability to manage cholesterol makes it an ideal food to take on any reducing diet. Lecithin capsules are inexpensive and available for those who prefer not to eat lecithin foods for fear of gaining weight. The better plan, it seems to me, is to take the lecithin capsules *and* eat foods rich in lecithin. Soybeans—rich in iron, calcium, and other minerals might well be one of the main foods on a weight watcher's diet.

Another food your heart will love is asparagus. Aspartic acid is one of the nonessential amino acids. Two French physicians, M. Lamarche and R. Royer, after animal experimentation, found that aspartic acid slows down the heart in a distress situation. What these Frenchmen did was to partially cut off the supply of oxygen to the heart causing it to beat faster and then introduce aspartic acid in the bloodstream, which caused a slowing down of beats per minute.

Other French doctors have found that aspartic acid decreases fatigue and increases available energy. They recommend that further studies be made to treat human coronary insufficiency with aspartic acid which they found was an important detoxifier. The mere fact that aspartic acid enables a heart to do its work on less oxygen is sufficient reason to add asparagus to the diet.

Nutrition experts Margaret and Ancel Keys, in a book, *The Benevolent Bean*, made a study of the relationship of the low coronary rate in Italy and the Italians' love of beans. An experiment was made with Minnesota men who ate, as Dr. Keys reported, "the leafy vegetables, the abundant fruits, the beans and other leguminous seeds so prominent in the daily diet of Naples." As a result, the cholesterol level of the Minnesotans fell from 225 to about 165, which is the average cholesterol reading of a Neapolitan.

In Roseto, a small Pennsylvania town largely inhabited by Italians, the rate of heart disease is so low that it set off a full-scale government-sponsored investigation of the diets and habits of those people, but the findings were inconclusive. Dr. Keys conducted other experiments using brown beans from Holland and peas from India. "If you happen to be interested in cholesterol control, beans or any leguminous seeds merit a prominent place in your diet," said Dr. Keys.

Americans are not big consumers of beans. If we ate a half pound of beans a week (the average Italian eats 82 grams of beans a day), it would double our intake of legumes. Dr. Keys further said: "Something else in the diet would have to be reduced to keep calories in line. Our proposal would be to reduce sugar. Nutritionally and gastronomically, too, it is scandalous that Americans get 16 per cent of their calories from sugar and other sweeteners. If we substituted 12 pounds of beans for an equal amount of sugar in the yearly diet, we would still be eating around 85 pounds of sugar a year."

Most of the foods we eat are good for the heart. Since heart attacks result from malnutrition, even when the victims are overweight, *any food* that is high in vitamins B, C, or E is beneficial to the heart. It is unfortunate that we cannot get all of the vitamins and minerals needed for healthy hearts from our daily food. When those vitamins and minerals have been processed out of the foods we buy, we *must* resort to vitamin and mineral supplements.

It is impossible for us to grow and mill grains in order to get the valuable and necessary nutrients our ancestors ate. Most of us don't have the time or the acreage to grow vegetable gardens. Fruit raising is out of the question with nearly everyone. So there is really no choice except to take the chance of coronary disease or protect ourselves with good nutrition. The instinct of self-preservation is strong enough with me that I go along with the "good nutrition" way. It has paid dividends in the kind of health I have—even at my age.

7 FOODS THAT ARE BAD FOR THE HEART

ABOUT A YEAR AGO I visited a friend in a hospital after a heart attack. He had been out of intensive care several days and was sitting up eating fruit upon which he poured three or four average servings of sugar. "Does your doctor allow you to eat sugar?" I asked. "Oh, yes, the only food I can't have is unsaturated fat. You know I have always been a big sugar eater." My friend never returned home—he died in the hospital from another heart attack.

On another occasion I visited a heart patient in a hospital who offered me some candy. I said, "No, thanks, I have a low blood sugar condition and I cannot eat any food that has sugar." My friend complained bitterly that his doctor would not permit him to have chocolate candy because it was "too fat." This friend did better than the one I first mentioned—he lived nearly a year after he left the hospital.

We all know that the great killers are the "diseases of civilization," diseases which might well be called the modern plagues of the western hemisphere and Europe. We also know that diabetes, ulcers, arthritis, cancers, and coronary diseases are either nonexistent or have a very low incidence rate in primitive countries. When sugar has been introduced into primitive countries, the disease and death rates have increased tremendously.

What is the principal cause of this fantastic plague

that is killing more people than all of the wars these so-called civilized people have engaged in this century? Could this misery and death have been avoided? My opinion is that refined sugar disables and kills millions of Americans every year. In *Mental Health Through Nutrition*, I showed how poor nutrition has filled our penal institutions with juvenile delinquents and criminals. In other books I have explained how poor nutritional habits are responsible for the breakdown of home life and the high divorce rate in the United States.

While this book relates to the causes of cardiovascular diseases and how such diseases can be avoided, the casual reader has already observed that we are talking about one big disease of modern civilization–malnutrition. When I speak of malnutrition I am not thinking of it in the same way as the politician who talks about hungry people, or as the physician who contends that if one gets enough food he cannot possibly be malnourished.

Dr. K. J. Kingsbury of St. Mary's Hospital had an article in *The Lancet* for December 24, 1966. He had conducted an extensive examination of 338 atherosclerotic male patients, mostly from London–from a complex group as far as social, economic, and occupational grounds are concerned. None of the men had diabetes. Dr. Kingsbury found that the intolerance to sugar was the cause of atherosclerosis and, the greater the degree of atherosclerosis, the less able was the subject to metabolize sugar.

Dr. Peter Kuo of the University of Pennsylvania, according to *Medical Tribune* (September 11, 1969), told the American Medical Association, meeting in New York, that the first approach to a therapy for atherosclerotic patients was the complete elimination of sugar and sugar-containing foods. Dr. Kuo said that complex carbohydrates, as whole wheat and potatoes, could be taken in limited amounts.

Dr. Kuo had studied 184 atherosclerotic patients. After years of investigation, he concluded that sugar and not fat is the culprit to be avoided to prevent and treat heart disease. Another interesting result from Dr. Kuo was that 166 of the 184 atherosclerotic patients studied lost weight on the sugar-restricted diets, most of them having lost more than fifteen pounds each.

Drs. Willard A. Krehl and Robert L. Hodges and associates of the University of Iowa, in an article in the November 1967 issue of the *American Journal of Clinical Nutrition*, reviewed the dietary conditions of people living in the western world, and concluded that the development of atherosclerotic heart disease resulted from the switch from the consumption of complex carbohydrates—as cereals, potatoes, and vegetables—to refined sugar and foods containing sugar.

These Iowa physicians had an article in the February 1967 *American Journal of Clinical Nutrition*, in which they stated: "As the amount of sucrose (refined sugar, etc.) is increased, and the quantity of complex cereals decreased, the concentration of cholesterol, and more particularly triglycerides, rises."

A survey of sixteen countries made by the Interdepartment Committee on Nutrition for National Development showed that the countries having the highest cholesterol readings also had the highest consumption of refined sugar.

In the book *Diet and Disease* by Dr. E. Cheraskin and others from the University of Alabama, the authors concluded that sugar increases the blood cholesterol while complex carbohydrates reduce the amount of cholesterol in the blood.

Dr. John Yudkin, one of the world's greatest nutritionists, in the July 4, 1964, issue of *The Lancet*, after years of study and research at the University of London, declared that sugar and not fat is the cause of atherosclerosis and heart attacks. Later, in answer to those who claimed that it was fat and not sugar that caused atherosclerosis, Dr. Yudkin showed that when people improved economically and ate more fat they always had increased sugar consumption in pies, cakes, and other fat foods. Dr. Yudkin asked two questions that cannot be answered by those who exonerate sugar and put the blame for heart disease on fats:

1. Why didn't our ancestors drop dead on all sides of heart attacks when they ate as much fat in their diets as we eat now?

2. Why should the incidence of heart disease have increased so sharply in modern times and keep growing from year to year?

Dr. T. R. Van Dellen, in his syndicated column *How to Keep Well* (copyright 1970 by *The Chicago Tribune*), said: "Some of the dangers associated with consuming . . . sugar are dental caries, arteriosclerosis and obesity, assuming you do not have diabetes."

The Nobel Prize in Medicine for 1964 was for a study demonstrating that the liver manufactures the cholesterol that goes into the blood out of acetic acid. One food, glucose, a common form of sugar, is entirely transformed into acetic acid in the course of body chemistry. The greatest dietary source of glucose is refined sugar. Since cholesterol is synthesized from acetic acid, if blood cholesterol is to be lowered, sugar must be eliminated from the diet.

Dr. Benjamin P. Sandler wrote, in his book, *How to Prevent Heart Attacks*, that it is sugar and not fats that cause atherosclerosis. Dr. Sandler said: "The Eskimo living within the Arctic Circle is notoriously free of arteriosclerosis and heart attacks, yet consumes an extremely high-fat diet compared with the average diet of Americans in the United States."

The October 12, 1963, issue of the *Canadian Medical Association Journal* noted that two pounds of sugar every week was consumed by each person in Britain and "that was the amount of sugar our . . . ancestors ate in a year." In 1965 Dr. Clifford Anderson, a California physician, said that a study of the eating habits of victims of heart attack showed they had been eating an average of 4.5 ounces of sugar daily while a control group of healthy men ate an average of 2.75 ounces of sugar each day. Dr. Anderson told physicians if they wanted to know the cause of heart disease to "take a close look at the sugar bowl."

A. S. Loginov had an article in a 1962 Russian heart journal, *Kardiologiya*, showing that the Ethiopians have a high fat diet, but practically no heart disease. A. M. Cohen, in a 1963 issue of the *American Heart Journal*, stated that Jews living in Yemen who ate very high fat diets had no heart disease, while those who migrated to Israel and ate a "civilized" diet had the same tendency to atherosclerosis evident in the United States and Western Europe.

Dr. T. L. Cleave, former Surgeon Captain of the Royal Navy of Great Britain, writing in the July 25, 1964, issue of *The Lancet*, indicted both refined sugar and refined flour as causes of heart disease.

The American people have been "sold a bill of goods" by the sugar trust. We do *not* have to eat sugar to get energy. To me sugar is a form of poison that starts to work as soon as we take it into our mouths by helping destroy our teeth.

Fifty years ago no one had ever heard of a child dying from heart disease except from infrequent rheumatic fever. In the last twenty to thirty years, an increasing and alarming number of young people die from coronary diseases.

A new textbook by Dr. Benjamin Gasul and associates, *Heart Disease in Children*, stated that what was formerly considered a degenerative disease of the middle-aged and elderly is rapidly becoming common among the very young.

Dr. Gasul, a prominent pediatrician, believes that hypertension is often unrecognized for many, many years. We know that salt and sugar cause hypertension, or high blood pressure. Infants and small children are frequently fed a diet high in sugar. Many infant formulas are loaded with sugar.

Dr. Lewis Dahl of the Medical Research Center of Brookhaven National Laboratory found that today's baby foods have a high salt content. He also noted that canned baby food fruits have sugary syrups added.

Dr. Dahl tested young rats to see what high salt intake would do. "Such rats are much more prone to develop hypertension than older animals," said Dr. Dahl. "In man it seems warranted to give serious consideration to the possibility that a high intake of sodium chloride might play an important part in the propagation of hypertension in adults," he continued.

Dr. Gasul noted that cow's milk has four times as much salt as human milk. He warned against the giving of any salted foods to infants who are on cow's milk. After observing that cow's milk is low in iron, Dr. Gasul said: "Chronic severe anemia may give rise to congestive heart failure. This is likely to be observed in children with iron-deficiency anemia of long standing."

When we look around and see what our youngsters are eating and drinking, we wonder how any of them can escape heart attacks when they are middle-aged or older. Sugar-coated cereals for breakfast, sugared soft drinks, candies, ice creams, hamburgers, and hot dogs—with practically no foods containing valuable vitamins and minerals—make up most of the diet of a majority of our teenagers.

I appreciate the difficulty parents have in eliminating from the diet of their children foods that are high in sugar, salt, and fat. All informed nutritionists agree that sugar, in combination with salt, causes hypertension much faster than does salt or sugar alone. I am certain that if parents knew that salt, sugar, and fats were involved in diseases of the heart, they would not be so indulgent with infants and young children with these dangerous foods.

Many medical writers have noted that in Britain during World War II, when stress was greater than usual, but sugar was rationed and difficult to get, the rate of heart deaths declined tremendously.

Researchers have been telling us for years that sugar destroys vitamins, particularly the B vitamins in our bodies. Sugar consumption increases by leaps and bounds every year and so do cardiovascular diseases. The average American eats considerably more than two pounds of sugar each week. When we consider the diabetics, the hypoglycemics, the dieters who have reduced sugar intake to control weight, and small children who cannot possibly eat two or three pounds of sugar every week, we can understand how a heavy user of sugar and sweetened foods eats the equivalent of four or five pounds of sugar in a week's time. How much proof will the medical profession require before it admits that sugar is not good for us?

After some physicians demonstrated that polyunsaturated fat without adequate intake of vitamin E caused so many serious and sometimes fatal diseases, one would think that all cardiologists would consider giving vitamin E to their patients. Blind medical prejudice should not result in hundreds of thousands of Americans being disabled and dying prematurely every year when vitamin and mineral supplementation could prevent all of that.

The difficulty with the saturated fat versus the unsaturated fat theories, as well as the theories regarding the causes and effects of high blood cholesterol levels, is that medical articles written in newspapers and magazines have been so contradictory or vague that most laymen are not informed, but are badly confused by what they read. When the American Heart Association came out in 1961 with a written report for laymen, which in part read: "Evidence gathered from many countries suggests a relationship between the amount and type of fat consumed, the amount of cholesterol in the blood and the reported incidence of coronary artery disease," the reader was not certain that animal fats caused heart disease or that unsaturated fats prevented coronary attacks.

Most of us assume that when we eat natural vegetables oils—as corn, cotton, soya and the like—we are getting polyunsaturated fats. The American Heart Association report of 1961 told us that "margarines have less than half as much saturated fat [as butter], and the common vegetable oils have still less." I am sure that 90 percent of those who use margarines and vegetable oils believe they are getting no saturated fats, which is not true.

Dr. Jackson Blair, a member of the medical staffs of several Cleveland hospitals, wrote in the August 1955 *Ohio State Medical Journal* that table mustard is a cause of coronary heart disease, arteriosclerosis, and high blood pressure. He also said that pepper and ginger can cause high blood pressure. Dr. Blair lists twelve cases he had observed where young and middle-aged users of mustard suffered coronary attacks.

When heart specialists disagree about what foods are bad for the heart, some contending that sugar and salt are not harmful and that we need only be concerned with saturated fats, while others take the opposite view, from a practical standpoint, we laymen need not become involved in such academic questions because fats, sugar, and salt usually go hand in hand. What I am trying to say is that the big sugar user who thinks he has to have pies, cakes, doughnuts, and the like, will eat a lot of fat and salt and be in trouble with his cholesterol regardless of what the heart specialists believe.

8 MINERALS AND HEART DISEASE

We know that with arteriosclerosis our arteries lose their ability to stretch; they become thick, brittle, and inflamed. With atherosclerosis plaques adhere to defects in the artery walls. If the plaques become large enough, the blood vessel is blocked and blood does not get to the heart or brain. The plaque may break loose and lodge in the heart causing coronary thrombosis.

The plaque is made up of cholesterol, calcium, and clotted blood. The first thought is, naturally, that if we want to avoid plaques we must eat less calcium foods, just as we are told to reduce our cholesterol foods to prevent atherosclerosis. Medical authorities generally agree that removing calcium from the diet promotes heart disease. It has been shown that extra calcium actually helps reduce heart disease by lowering cholesterol levels.

The British Medical Journal for May 22, 1965, reported several cases where the subjects had been given supplementary calcium. Cholesterol blood levels dropped in all of those so tested.

On July 10, 1965, a New Jersey medical research team composed of Drs. Marvin Bierenbaum, Alan Fleischman, and H. Yacowitz observed that extensive experiments with persons who had never had heart disease showed lower blood serum cholesterol after increased calcium intake.

Drs. J. N. Morris, M. D. Crawford, and J. A. Heady, British medical researchers at London Hospital medical school, found that the calcium of hard water inhibited heart attacks while the sodium of soft water increased death rates from heart disease. Dr. Henry Schroeder of Dartmouth University medical school found that parts of the central states with hard water had fewer heart disease deaths than did some coastal states with soft water.

Drs. M. J. Gardner and associates reported in the April 20, 1968, issue of *The Lancet* that a study of sixty-one English towns showed lower death rates in those with hard water than in the towns with soft water.

On April 14, 1965, Dr. Barry Fanburg, a Boston heart specialist, gave a technical paper at the annual meeting of the Federation of American Societies for Experimental Biology on how calcium affects the heart and why it is indispensable to the heart. The paper is too technical to attempt to give in detail, but Dr. Fanburg's conclusions may be summarized as follows: first, there must be an ample amount of calcium in the body for the heart to circulate blood through the body at all times and under all conditions; second, calcium is essential for regular heartbeats; and, third, calcium is responsible for the ability of the heart to relax between heartbeats.

At a meeting of the society mentioned in the preceding paragraph in April 1969, Drs. Bierenbaum and Fleischman presented proof from experiments with subjects with high blood levels of cholesterol and triglycerides that calcium caused a decrease in the cholesterol and triglyceride blood levels in such persons.

Scientists are not certain how calcium lowers cholesterol and triglyceride levels. It has been suggested that calcium forces the fats from the bloodstream and that they are eliminated as wastes instead of being absorbed into body tissues.

Dr. H. C. Sherman in his book *Calcium and Phosphorus* states that there is much evidence that we, in the western hemisphere, may be deficient in calcium. Most nutritionists believe that while our diet may be lacking in calcium, we may be getting too much phosphorus for the amount of calcium ingested. All authorities agree that unless we have an adequate amount of phosphorus in the diet, calcium will be excreted from the body unused. The ideal amount of calcium is two and one half times as much calcium as phosphorus.

We must have vitamin D for calcium and phosphorus to be absorbed. Nature has provided us with vitamin D from sunshine but most of us cannot, and should not, expose our bodies to sunlight to get the needed vitamin D. We hear a lot about vitamin D poisoning. I have asked a number of doctors if they had ever seen a case of vitamin D poisoning and all of them said "no," but mentioned that they had read of such cases.

Vitamin D in excessive amounts is toxic, but the amount of vitamin D that is injurious to an adult is higher than most physicians believe it to be. Actually, under federal law, your druggist cannot sell you a vitamin D capsule or tablet that has enough vitamin D in it to harm you. Many men and women have told me that they have taken 4,000 units of vitamin D daily for years with no toxic effects. I have taken 2,000 units of vitamin D each day for years—in fact, I do not absorb calcium and phosphorus with less than 2,000 units of vitamin D.

Vitamin A also helps the absorption of minerals. It, too, can be toxic if taken in excessive amounts.

I have read of men and women who have taken 100,000 units of vitamin A daily for years with no adverse side results, but I would not recommend that anyone take that amount. I take 25,000 units of vitamin A daily and that seems to be the amount recommended by physicians who have taken the time to learn something about vitamin and mineral supplementation in the diet. Many people have told me they regularly take 50,000 units of vitamin A each day with no toxic effects.

My preference for calcium is bone meal tablets which I take with each meal. I also drink milk which is an excellent source of calcium and phosphorus. Primitive men ate the bones of animals, which we cannot do. Bone meal, manufactured from the bones of young beef cattle, contains all of the minerals our bodies require and in exactly the right proportions.

Stroke is the third leading cause of death in this country, outranked only by heart disease and cancer. The usual cause of stroke is cerebral thrombosis, the formation of a blood clot on an artery that has been narrowed by cholesterol deposits. Persons with high blood pressure are the ones who have strokes most often.

Experiments conducted on rats show that calcium deficiency will cause strokes. Reports from researchers in America and abroad indicate that a diet high in calcium and low in salt may help protect the body from arteriosclerosis. Much effort is being made to rehabilitate stroke patients, but very little has been done in the United States to try to prevent this crippling and killing disease.

Any dietary program that helps prevent the accumulation of plaques on the arterial walls will go a long way toward preventing strokes. Waiting until the patient has a stroke and then treating him with medication sounds too much like waiting for the storm to hit before fixing the roof of a building.

Dr. Winifred Nayler of Baker Medical Research told us in the March 1967 issue of *Heart Journal* that calcium, while fundamentally necessary to the heartbeat, must have a sufficient quantity of magnesium in the body to be effective.

Dr. R. H. Seller, in the *Journal of the American Medical Association* for February 22, 1965, explained that magnesium induces the muscles of the circulatory system to relax and thus lowers high blood pressure. Dr. Mildred Seelig in the June 1964 *American Journal of Clinical Nutrition* found that there was a direct relation between the amount of magnesium in the diet and the avoidance of high blood pressure. Dr. Seelig estimated that the average American diet falls short about 200 milligrams a day (sometimes more) the optimal amount of magnesium one needs for good health.

A British research team produced evidence that drinking hard water offers protection against heart disease, reported *The Lancet* on February 4, 1967. These scientists found that the calcium and magnesium content of hard water "is of importance in relation to the concentration of these elements in the tissues."

G. E. Bunce and associates at Fitzsimmons General Hospital in the August 1965 *Journal of Nutrition* found that kidney stone formation was caused by magnesium deficiency. Other researchers have reported that when magnesium is deficient, excesses of calcium and phosphorus can no longer be eliminated, but are deposited upon vital tissues as the heart, liver, and kidneys.

Magnesium oxide is an excellent form of dietary magnesium. Magnesium is a mild laxative so one must be careful of the amount of magnesium taken. As the science of biochemistry becomes more advanced, we know more and more how important magnesium is to our good health. Until recent years magnesium and most of the trace minerals were considered unimportant to heart health.

Potassium is another mineral that is essential to the health of the heart. In some unknown way a duel seems to be fought in the body between sodium (salt) and potassium. When salt seems to win, the supply of potassium in the body is low; when potassium predominates, the amount of bodily salt is reduced.

Dr. Samuel Bellet in his book, *Potassium; Cardiac Aspects, the Role of Potassium in Health and Disease*, reported: "Animals fed diets low in potassium failed to grow at a normal rate. After several weeks the heart shows evidence of myocardial necrosis . . . a heart lesion may be produced in four days by a diet low in potassium and high in sodium chloride, together with injections of desoxycorticosterone-acetate."

Researchers have shown that countries with diets rich in potassium have a much lower rate of heart disease deaths than do countries with low-potassium diets. In the *New York State Journal of Medicine* for June 15, 1957, Drs. J. Yerushalmy and Herman Hilleboe presented evidence from many countries that greater consumption of fats did not increase the mortality rate for deaths from heart ailments. These scientists showed that in countries whose fat consumption was the same as ours, but whose people ate a richer potassium diet than in the United States, the mortality rate for heart diseases was slightly over one third that in this nation.

Dr. W. A. Krehl, in *Nutrition in Clinical Medicine* (June 22, 1966), said: "If food habits had always been sound, the event of potassium deficiency and depletion would not have developed as a major medical problem."

Zinc, according to Dr. Walter J. Pories of the University of Rochester, is important to a healthy heart. He found that all patients tested who had atherosclerosis had low zinc values. Other investigators in this country and abroad have uniformly found that atherosclerotic patients have low zinc levels.

We know that if the theory of many physicians as to the cause of coronary thrombosis is correct and the disease is not the result of food and mineral deficiencies, it would be evenly distributed across the United

States in proportion to the aging population. Large geographic differences in the death rates from cardiovascular diseases exist in our own country, which cannot be explained by the "unsaturated fats and stress" theories.

As Dr. Pories has said, cardiac death rates are higher in those parts of the United States with high water drainage, as where the minerals have been washed into rivers, the Gulf of Mexico, and the Great Lakes. It has been shown that 32 of the 50 states are zinc deficient.

The effective role of zinc in helping heal arterial lesions and the weight of evidence showing that coronary thrombosis is more of an environmental problem than a degenerative disease, indicate that mineral imbalance plays a big role in causing all cardiovascular diseases.

Chromium is another mineral helpful in maintaining proper cholesterol levels. Dr. Henry A. Schroeder has shown that chromium-fed rats have low cholesterol levels while chromium deficient animals have high levels of cholesterol. Scientists have determined that we are born with high tissue levels of chromium, but the amount declines as we grow older. In countries where chromium levels are high, hardening of the arteries and diabetes are seldom found.

Rats deprived of chromium developed diabetes and atherosclerosis, while rats fed chromium lived longer and were free of diabetes and circulatory diseases. Dr. Schroeder showed that the more sugar one eats the greater is his need for chromium. As Dr. Schroeder has pointed out, wheat, before the minerals are lost in milling, is our best source of chromium.

Vanadium, one of the trace minerals, is important to cardiovascular health. Researchers have found that, where drinking water has an abundance of vanadium, death rates from degenerative heart disease are low. In the soft water areas of the Great Lakes states and the coastal areas where vanadium is deficient in the water, heart death rates are highest.

Sea fish are an excellent source of this mineral. The low incidence of death from heart disease in the Scandinavian countries is attributed to the fish-eating habit of the Scandinavians. Meats are low in vanadium as are most vegetables. You will be doing your heart a favor when you eat ocean fish which contains other necessary minerals and valuable vitamins.

Copper in insufficient amount in the body leads to weakened blood vessels. The amount of copper required for health is very small. Earl Frieden in the May 1968 *Scientific American* showed that copper deficiency may cause the aorta (the large artery leading from the heart) to be susceptible to aneurysm and rupture. Liver, heart, brains, seafoods, and yeast are excellent sources of copper.

The other trace minerals—particularly manganese, cobalt, and molybdenum—as well as iron are essential to heart health. It is believed that bone meal supplements are the cheapest source of minerals available to us. The British medical journal, *The Lancet*, pointed out on May 14, 1966 that practically nothing is known about the role of some trace minerals in nutrition and about everything is yet to be learned about them. The editorial predicted that increased knowledge of trace minerals will have an impact comparable to that of vitamins.

As *The Lancet* editorial stated, much study has been made of a few minerals by nutritional researchers, but we have no appreciable body of knowledge about mineral nutrition. The entire field of mineral nutritional knowledge is a virgin wilderness waiting to be explored. The editorial concluded that leading British nutritional doctors—and undoubtedly those in America—know so little about mineral nutrition that no one can begin to say which trace minerals are, or are not, essential.

9 NUTRITION AND BLOOD PRESSURE

WHEN YOUR BLOOD pressure is abnormally high, you are twice as likely to have a stroke or a heart attack. High blood pressure is nature's way of turning on a warning light of impeding danger. That is why your doctor keeps such a careful check on your blood pressure.

Physicians generally refer to high blood pressure as hypertension and when no known cause exists it is called "essential hypertension." Hypertension usually shows up when we are between thirty and fifty years old. It will not, in and of itself, kill or maim you for life. Its danger is that it may lead to heart disease, cerebral hemorrhage, or several other dreaded diseases.

Doctors tell us we should expect the blood pressure to be higher as we grow older, but I think high blood pressure, like senility, is something that can be avoided in old age. My blood pressure at 76 was exactly what it was when I was 30 years old.

There are many causes of high blood pressure. Your doctor will usually tell you to take off weight, leave salt out of your diet as much as possible, and get more exercise. He couldn't give you any better advice as far as it goes. But will he explain to you how you can get the blood pressure back to normal, and keep it that way with harmless nutrition? Will he and you try to take the easy course of correcting your hypertension with drugs?

In the *Journal of the American Medical Association* for October 6, 1969, Dr. Alvin P. Shapiro of the University of Pittsburgh medical school, in answer to a question whether a 36-year-old man who has suffered high blood pressure for eighteen years should be given drugs, said: "Our own policy is not to give specific hypotensive medications to such patients; the occurrence of side effects of long term therapy with the thiazides, for instance, which include gout, hyperglycemia and hypokalemia, is frequent. . . ."

Again in the February 9, 1970, issue of the *Journal of the American Medical Association*, Dr. S. K. Robinson, an Indiana physician, stressed the importance of always bringing down high blood pressure, but in a patient with long-term hypertension, by bringing the pressure down with nonmedical methods if possible, rather than by resorting to drugs. Dr. Robinson cites figures from Metropolitan Life Insurance Company and others to show that a young man with a blood pressure of 140 over 90 to 150 over 100 (as compared to one with a normal blood pressure of 125 over 80) is eight times more apt to have a coronary heart attack or a stroke.

We all know that high blood pressure makes the heart work harder to force the blood out into circulation against higher resistance. This means abnormal wear and tear on the blood vessels and the heart.

Studies by scientists of various countries where hypertension is not a problem have indicated that the people were low salt eaters. In America it was found that those whose salt intake was high were usually the ones with high blood pressure.

Nutritionists know of the importance of vitamins A, B, C, and E in reducing blood pressure. A pamphlet put out by the National Heart Institute in 1969, *Hypertension*, gave this advice: "Almost all cases of hypertension, whether mild or very severe, can be controlled by any of a variety of effective drugs or combination of drugs for reducing elevated blood pressure."

Since all that drugs can do is to *control* high blood pressure, wouldn't it be more scientific to get at the cause of hypertension, if at all possible, with the use of harmless foods and minerals? Why run the risk of dangerous side effects from the drugs–gout, ulcers, diabetes, gastrointestinal diseases, and so on–without giving nutrition a chance? Medication is so simple and easy–just give the nation's 17 to 32 million suffering high blood pressure drugs to control hypertension! Do the benefits to the millions of people who take drugs to reduce high blood pressure outweigh the dangerous side effects from the drugs? Certainly the most optimistic drug manufacturer would not contend that prescribed drugs have slowed down, much less stopped, the ever increasing death and disability rates from cardiovascular diseases.

The thiazide type of drugs force the kidneys to excrete salt and thus reduce blood pressure. Since a low-salt diet will do what the drug does, why should anyone take the medication? I think the answer is found in the ease with which a doctor can write a prescription and the time it will take to explain to the patient why a low-salt diet is required. Most patients are looking for "wonder drugs" which they never find.

Instead of having National Heart Days, we should have National Vitamin E Days or National Nutrition Days. We know that people who are able to keep their blood pressure at healthy levels live longer than those with high blood pressure.

A diet high in sugar and saturated fats was cited by Dr. Robinson as related to high blood pressure. There is one point upon which all physicians agree; weight reduction has the greatest and most lasting effect on lowering blood pressure.

When blood pressure is *very high,* all nutritionists agree that drugs, diet, vitamin, and mineral supplements and reasonable exercise should be used. Time is too important to waste with experimentation with a patient who may have a stroke or heart attack any time.

In a Canadian study reported in the *Journal of the American Geriatrics Society* for August 28, 1968, it was said that the mortality rate for those whose high blood pressure has been brought down to normal was about half the rate for those not treated.

Dr. W. W. Priddle and associates told a medical group in Toronto that, of 183 patients having a systolic blood pressure of 180 or over and a diastolic blood pressure of 100 or more, 100 were treated and blood pressures lowered. Later, it was found of the 100 who accepted treatment only 29 had died, while of the 83 who were not treated 49 had died.

Dr. Otto Schaeffer, who lived among the Eskimos for several years and had examined the blood pressure of more than four thousand Eskimos, found that high blood pressure and bad hearts do not exist among

Eskimos under 60 years old and are far less common in old Eskimos than in elderly whites. Dr. Schaeffer believes that the reason for this is the Eskimos' aversion to salted food.

Dr. Lewis K. Dahl reported on salt usage and high blood pressure in the June 5 and 12, 1959, issues of the *New England Journal of Medicine*. In northern Japan, where the salt intake is higher than in southern Japan, deaths from brain hemorrhages are much greater. In America, Dr. Dahl said, the tissues of stroke victims showed a much higher salt content than did the tissues of those who died from other causes.

Dr. Dahl said that his patients complained for a week or so about the taste of food after salt had been eliminated from their diets. He emphasized that salt appetite is acquired and not a basic need. "Salt appetite is not to be equated with salt requirement," said Dr. Dahl.

When the blood pressure is high, it is best to eat as little salt as possible. Those of us who do not have high blood pressure should use the salt shaker "hardly at all."

Dr. Dahl suggested that people who have a family history of high blood pressure should drastically reduce the amount of salt eaten and increase the amount of potassium foods in the diet to offset the salt consumed. People are fortunate who like tomato catsup because of its high potassium content. I was sitting at a table in a restaurant with a couple recently when the wife complained that her husband ruined the taste of everything good with tomato catsup. I couldn't help saying, "It may keep him from having a heart attack."

Francisco R. Jose and associates found a close relationship between the amounts of salt eaten and cholesterol levels. These Philippine scientists fed salt to young rats, resulting in slower growth and increased blood and liver cholesterol.

Dr. William E. Morton of the University of Oregon made an extensive study of the effects of nitrites and nitrates on blood pressure. He reported that in a certain area in Colorado where hypertension was general the concentration of nitrate was heavy. He cited other evidence from research laboratories indicating "that long-acting organic nitrates might hasten the progress of coronary artery disease rather than alleviate it." Dr. Morton referred to findings from other countries that exposure to nitrates produced "chronic cardiovascular toxic effects."

We know that nitrates are excessively used in agriculture for fertilization and that some plants have concentrations of nitrates far in excess of a safe level for food. Nitrous food additives have been added to foods we buy in our grocery stores.

We may be getting hypertension from chemicals in our foods and from the water we drink. The best way to fight the toxins from nitrates is to take vitamins B complex and C which have been proven to be antitoxic vitamins. Wouldn't it be wonderful if the food on the grocery store shelves carried this label, "No nitrates or nitrites!" We would then know that we were not buying high blood pressure.

If you have normal blood pressure and want to keep

it that way, you should hold your food intake down. Eliminate sweets and cut down on carbohydrates. If you stop salting your food on the table, it will not be long before you find that you like foods better without added salt.

Above all, as you grow older, don't take the fatalistic attitude that high blood pressure and overweight are inevitable. In 90 percent of the cases overweight and high blood pressure are the results of careless nutritional habits. Even among the 10 percent or less who develop "secondary hypertension," or high blood pressure as a result of some malfunctioning of the body, the condition can generally be successfully treated and cured.

The most important thing we can do to stay alive and be healthy is to keep the blood pressure normal.

10 WHAT CAN BE DONE ABOUT OBESITY

EVEN THOUGH MANY doctors readily admit that they know little or nothing about nutrition, every physician for the past fifty or seventy-five years has known that obesity is a killer. Excess weight harms the whole body, but it is the heart that is hurt the most.

Life insurance companies have told us recently that a man 45 years old who is 30 percent overweight can expect to die in 12 years, while a man of the same age with normal weight ordinarily has another 25 years ahead of him.

We are also told that an overweight man has three times the death rate from heart disease of an underweight man and twice the rate of death of one of normal weight. If you have high blood pressure and are obese, any doctor will tell you that if you want to live you have no other choice than to take off weight.

I think many physicians approach the obesity problem in the wrong manner. They tell their patients they must take off weight without telling them how to reduce. Most doctors are so obsessed with the term, "balanced diet," which they erroneously assume means eating everything, that they will not tell the patients what foods to stop eating.

A doctor will say to an overweight person with high blood pressure: "Salt and sugar are bad for the heart, so go on as nearly a salt-free and a sugar-free diet as you possibly can. Don't worry about salt; you get a lot of natural salt in your foods and salt has been added to most processed and manufactured foods. You will get all of the natural sugar you need from unsweetened fruits and vegetables. The body converts the proteins you eat into a form of blood sugar that is good for you."

No fat man wants to start counting calories so the wise doctor will say: "Stay with lean meats. You may have beef, pork, fish, chicken, turkey, or other fowls. Eat eggs at least every other day. Eat fruits, salads, and vegetables, but go easy on bread and potatoes. You should not eat fried foods. As you get accustomed to this diet, you will find that you like it and that you are taking smaller servings at each meal.

"Breakfast is your most important meal, so stop skipping breakfast. If you get hungry in the middle of the morning, or in the middle of the afternoon, eat something. You have been a long time putting on all that extra weight, so don't try to take it all off in a week or even in a month. The important thing about any diet is to stop stuffing yourself with sugars and other carbohydrates with little or no food value. You don't need to starve, or even feel empty, to take off weight. You do have to be selective about what you eat. The feeling of being alive and alert as the pounds melt away will more than compensate for anything you gave up to take off those extra pounds."

Most physicians believe that a woman during pregnancy should not be on a low-salt diet to prevent a gain in weight. If one has very low blood pressure, his doctor will usually advise him against reducing his salt intake.

The Michigan School of Public Health conducted a study of 746 male workers in 1962. Most of them were slim as young men and a majority were obese in middle age. Those who had not put on weight generally did not have high blood pressure. Blood pressure rose with the obese as weight increased.

Experiments conducted with overweight subjects in America and England showed that those who were called hypertensive (who had a blood pressure of 150 over 100 or more) had a reduction in blood pressure as they lost weight.

For years I was overweight. Now I weigh thirty pounds less than I did when I was 25 years old. For some time I have eaten three good meals a day. I don't eat the kind of foods that make me obese. I am never as hungry as I was most of the time when I was overweight.

We are fortunate that the damaging effects of obesity can be reversed when the excess weight is taken off. There is no time like *now* to start taking off those extra pounds. Most important, however, is when you start to lose weight, keep right on reducing until you reach the goal you have set for your weight.

Most women's magazines feature "crash diets." Overweight women try the "seven days," the "ten days," and the "fourteen days" reducing diets. One does take off a few pounds on a crash diet, then he or she goes on an eating binge and in three or four days is heavier than ever.

I appreciate the difficulties a housewife faces when she tries to lose weight. We men don't have to think about foods and we are not tempted to eat while preparing, planning, and serving meals as are our wives.

Many obese people are compulsive eaters. For years when I had an emotional problem I usually tried to solve it by an excessive amount of food. Now, when an emotional problem arises, I take a three- or four-mile walk which I have found helps get rid of what is "eating on me" better than over-doing with food.

Fortunately, most of those with emotional problems, instead of gorging on foods or taking tranquilizing drugs, engage in some community service work for their schools, churches, civic clubs, fraternal organizations, destitute and underprivileged children, and dozens of other worthwhile enterprises, which help dissolve emotional difficulties.

If you are one who eats excessively because of some unsolved personal problem, I recommend that you get your problem out in the open and, if you need professional help, see a minister, a lawyer, a marriage counselor, or other expert. Solving your emotional problems will generally take care of your excessive eating habit.

During my thirty years as a divorce trial judge, I was told by hundreds of men and women (more women than men) that they ate too much food because they were unhappy. They seemed to try to compensate for loneliness, feeling unloved and unwanted, thinking they were unworthy or inadequate, and they rebelled against cruelty and neglect by overindulging in food.

The principal reason for obesity is the same thing that causes most heart attacks: *malnutrition.* Somehow, if we are not getting the minerals and vitamins nature intended that we get, our bodies cry out for food even though we are dangerously overweight. When we start eating the vitamins, minerals, and other foods our bodies require for health and strength, our abnormal appetites become normal.

Most obese individuals take very little exercise largely because obesity makes them tired. Some have the erroneous impression that exercise increases the appetite and makes one heavier than if he remained idle. Look around you at those who are active physically. They are not obese. True, it does take a lot of exercise to burn up a pound of fat, but that isn't the point. Physical exercise makes one more trim, more firm, gets rid of body poisons, helps digestion, and improves general health, the net result of which is we no longer eat a lot of useless and needless foods. It may sound complex but it is simple to the nutritionist.

Dr. J. T. Keeve, New York health expert, wrote in the January 1965 *Journal of School Health*: "A chief reason for concern is the fact that juvenile obesity not only persists into adult life, but tends to be more severe and more difficult to treat than obesity occurring in adult life."

Dr. Hilda Bruch in her book, *The Importance of Overweight*, placed the blame for overweight children on mothers who could have prevented it while the child was very young. Dr. Bruch said that an infant would cry for some cuddling and comfort but the mother would thrust a bottle in the baby's mouth instead of holding him. Naturally, the baby linked the satisfaction of eating with his emotional needs, and the link between emotional satisfaction and food persisted as the child matured.

It has been estimated that we have more than 10 million children who are overweight. Physicians agree that being fat is a serious threat to both the physical and mental health of our children.

Mothers often appear to be trying to make "fatties" out of their babies by overfeeding them. They seem to be more interested in what the scales say about the infant's gain in weight than in his future health.

Dr. J. J. Oldfield, famous English nutritionist, in the October 5, 1968, *British Medical Journal*, placed some of the blame for the baby's overeating on his pediatrician. He said: "On every side we hear of the problem of the fat child who grows into the obese adult with all the well-known attendant hazards."

Other well-known physicians have warned mothers against the advice given by other mothers, doting relatives, and doctors that the child "will grow out of it," meaning that he will slender up as he grows older. These doctors report that these fat youngsters usually grow heavier.

Parents should realize that a fat child is an unhappy child, missing much of the fun of other children! He never has robust health, and as he gets older is forever trying "this and that" fad reducing diet, winding up with high blood pressure and all of the diseases that go with being too heavy.

Some mothers make bad matters worse by setting up a system of rewards of fattening foods for their children's good conduct. A mother should never forget that overweight is "from the cradle to the grave." She should be more concerned about developing a normal, healthy child than in trying to stuff a whole jar of mixed vegetables and meat into a few weeks' old baby.

Dr. Jean Mayer, Harvard nutritionist, stated in the February 1966 *Ladies Home Journal* that mothers exaggerate the importance of milk and that many children drink too much of it. Referring to sweets, Dr. Mayer said, "The great American dessert is a pernicious habit. If a child is brought up without it, he doesn't miss it."

Gussie Mason in her book, *How to Help Your Child Lose Weight*, said that if a mother permitted her child to get his own breakfast she could have no hope for his diet.

Mothers should always remember that their overweight children desperately need vitamins and minerals. The reducing foods for a child are substantially the same as those for an adult–avoid foods that are high in calories but low in nutrition. Most doctors recommend between-meal snacks for children.

One of the problems of the obese child is that he does not get the exercise necessary for growth and development. If you visit a school playground, you will observe that the fat children stand around and do not participate in the activities of other youngsters.

Dr. Jean Mayer and other nutritionists have found that obese children suffer severe psychological trauma resulting in personality traits similar to those observed by sociologists in oppressed minority groups who were victims of intense hatred. The obese child after maturity avoids challenges, has no independence, and is willing to settle for the humdrum.

Parents of obese children must early introduce them to the joys of physical activities and participation in athletics. These children must never be allowed to drift into a monotonous, sedentary life.

The important thing for the new mother to remember is that when a baby feels that he has his mother's love, support, and cooperation, he is not apt to take solace in calories he does not need and make useless weight.

11 EXERCISE IS GOOD FOR THE HEART

THE DEAN OF American cardiologists, Dr. Paul Dudley White, believes that vigorous exercise, begun early in life and steadily maintained, is one of the best things we can do to assure lifelong heart health. In the first of a number of syndicated articles in daily newspapers, Dr. White wrote: "My devotion to walking and bicycling has not been an accidental association. Rather it signifies my deep feeling of the importance of using the leg muscles as an integral part of the maintenance of a proper circulation, as well as a deterrent to cardiovascular disease."

The great Canadian cardiologist, Dr. Wilfrid E. Shute, has said: "Often the difference between life and death lies in the amount of collateral circulation to the heart that has been developed. It is only through exercise that the heart gains such an auxiliary blood and oxygen supply."

Forty years ago, when one had coronary thrombosis, his physician put him to bed for six weeks or longer. This is no longer the plan used by doctors. When the patient has made sufficient recovery to warrant it, his physician will have him resume such physical activity as the doctor feels may be safe.

Dr. Wilfred E. Shute reported that the new method of getting heart patients up in armchairs when chest pains were relieved has reduced the initial death rate to 9.9 percent as compared with the old rate of 40 to 60 percent of deaths with long bed rest.

Surgeons get patients up and moving around after serious surgery to prevent blood clotting and calcium depletion. Experiments with healthy young people forced to lie in beds with plaster casts showed that they soon started to excrete calcium in their urine, proving that calcium depletion results from a lack of exercise. Other experiments have shown that increased exercise requires increased amounts of calcium in the diet.

Dr. Jean Mayer, Harvard University nutritionist, in the December 1966 issue of *Clinical Nutrition*, stated that much of our soaring disease rate can be traced to a lack of exercise. He cited heart disease, diabetes, and osteoporosis as partly resulting from our sedentary lives. "It may well be that no currently available medical measure could be as beneficial as an increase in the amount of exercise taken by our population "

Drs. Samuel M. Fox, III, and James S. Skinner, in an article in the December 1964 *American Journal of Cardiology*, said: "Concurrent with a reduction in the requirements for physical activity in modern living, there has been an increase in death and disability from cardiovascular diseases." These researchers told of experiments in over two hundred hospitals with these results: "Physical activity of work is a protection against coronary (ischemic) heart disease. . . . Regular physical exercise could be one of the 'ways of life' that promote health in middle age."

Dr. George Mann in an article published December

25, 1965, in *The Lancet* described the Masai tribe in Tanzania, who have low blood pressure, healthy arteries, and low cholesterol levels. They are a fat-eating people who eat no sugar or other refined carbohydrates, no salt, and few vegetables. They walk great distances every day which seems to lower cholesterol levels and clear plaques from the arteries. Dr. Mann concluded that "coronary-heart disease, obesity and diabetes, the prevalent chronic diseases of Western Society, are a consequence of . . . indolence and inactivity."

Of all forms of exercise that benefit the heart, walking is perhaps best. Most Americans take very little exercise, preferring to use an automobile instead of walking a block or so to mail a letter or run some other errand. Those who do walk may prevent a fatal heart attack.

Most of us after a heavy meal prefer to take a nap instead of a short walk. In so doing we may be inviting a tragedy. Dr. Gerhard Volkheimer of Humboldt University medical school (Germany), in *Food and Nutrition News* for January 1965, said that napping after a heavy meal may lead to a fatal heart attack.

According to the May 24, 1965, *Medical Tribune*, Dr. Herman Hellerstein of Cleveland does six miles of walking daily. Dr. Hellerstein's treatment for heart patients is diet, no smoking, and gradual exercise as strength increases. His patients avoid elevators, climb stairs, and park their cars and walk part way to and from work.

Dr. Joseph B. Wolffe, medical director of the Valley Forge Medical Center and Heart Hospital, speaking before the 44th Annual National Recreation Congress in Philadelphia, stated:

"My presentation is from a heart specialist's point of view, although you doubtlessly would hear similar observations from a rheumatologist, orthopedic surgeon, or a neurologist.

"Leading cardiologists—both clinicians and researchers—of the American Heart Association and the National Health Institute are in agreement that one of the factors contributing to atherosclerosis is lack of exercise. Atherosclerosis, widely prevalent disease of Western civilization and the most common form of 'hardening of the arteries,' is often regarded as a degenerative disease due to aging. While age is a factor, there are many old people in our country and vast numbers in countries like Yemen and parts of Africa and China, who are comparatively free from this disease.

"Atherosclerosis is characterized by accumulation of cholesterol and other fatty debris in the walls of the medium and large-sized arteries which often plug the lumen, thus impeding or blocking the flow of blood. . . . In a study conducted at the Valley Forge Medical Center and Heart Hospital, we were impressed by a lack of clinical and laboratory evidence of atherosclerosis in a group of outstanding athletes who were continuing strenuous athletic endeavor well into their advancing years. Among them were old marathon runners up to 67 years old. The cardiovascular efficiency of these active individuals was far superior to a comparative group of executives of a leading industrial firm of similar age level. This study confirms

Mellerowicz's finding that the cardiovascular systems of old athletes who continued regular training were functionally equivalent to those of a much younger age group of the average population. . . .

"In a survey by Pomeroy and White, favorable results were reported on the influence of lifelong exercise in their study of ex-football players. Those who maintained a heavy exercise program throughout the postplaying years did not develop coronary heart disease. A study by Morris and his group in Great Britain showed that the number of heart attacks among sedentary workers, clerks, switchboard operators and truck drivers was three times greater than among those engaged in physically active occupations—laborers, miners, transport workers and farmers.

"The term 'athlete's heart,' which unfortunately still carries a connotation of abnormalcy, is a myth. There is no such clinical entity . . . It is important to caution here that individuals who are not accustomed to vigorous physical activity, or who have not exercised for a long time, should not indulge in strenuous physical effort without preparation. The man who has a heart attack while shoveling snow, whose only exercise prior to this vigorous exercise (since snow is heavy) was pushing a pen, a button, picking up a telephone receiver, or driving his car, only proves that he was 'soft.' His coronary arteries did not respond to a sudden need for meeting his unaccustomed demand. Many individuals are in very poor physical condition, but recreational exercise would condition them, reeducate their muscles, and reduce the number of heart attacks as well as sudden deaths.

"The staff of the Valley Forge Medical Center and Heart Hospital insisted for more than a decade that there should be no elevator for their own or the patients' use. It is a three-story building. Eighty-five per cent of the patients suffer from either cardiac or vascular disease or both. Patients with acute heart failure or acute coronary thrombosis who should be at complete bed rest for a limited period are placed on the first floor. However, as soon as these patients are ambulatory and have been rehabilitated, they are encouraged to walk stairs.

"Stair walking involves all systems in the body. The body is carried upward by the skeletal muscles. Groups of muscles contract while their antagonists relax. . . . The heart and vessels are gradually strengthened. . . . One can walk at a pace which does not produce shortness of breath resulting from oxygen debt. . . . The nervous system plays its part in stair walking. The afferent and efferent nerves are flashing out impulses to improve the individual's coordination. . . .

"The endocrine system also plays a part even during such mild exercise as walking stairs. More corticosteroids are excreted at this time–these are the hormones that are used in the treatment of arthritis. This is another proof that physical movements are essential for the arthritic patient. . . .

"In all the years of my medical practice, I have yet to see any patient with heart disease die while walking stairs. I have known hundreds who died in bed. . . . The person–unless he is crippled–who avoids walking steps fails to take advantage of a safe 'built-in exercise.' I would exchange many fancy pills and injectable wonder drugs for a hospital recreation expert who would recondition or recreate these individuals whose bodies are wrecked as the result of the monotonous humdrum of life, the confinement indoors, and the lack of recreational activity."

(With permission from Alice K. Hand, administratrix of the estate of Joseph B. Wolffe and Valley Forge Medical Center and Heart Hospital, Norristown, Pennsylvania.)

The Germans walk more than do the people of the United States. The German death rate from heart disease is much lower than it is in this nation, showing that exercise does prevent degenerative heart disease.

Walking is the easiest and most inexpensive way to exercise. It can be varied to suit our strength and needs. At a meeting in Toronto in October 1966, sponsored by the Canadian Medical Association and attended by famous cardiologists from all over the world, it was found that exercise for the heart is not a fad but finds support in an enormous body of medical research. The symposium said that what was considered dubious a few years ago is rapidly becoming an irrefutable fact—that is, exercise is good for the heart. Even after a heart attack, these famous physicians said, sensible exercise will benefit the heart. These men said that the heart, like all other muscles, becomes stronger as we exercise it more and place greater demands on it. When the heart is not exercised, its muscle tissue degenerates and shrinks away making the heart vulnerable to disease.

What I have just reported is not new. Dr. Paul

Dudley White and other cardiologists have been telling us the same thing for years. If the heart is damaged or the general health is bad, one should exercise, particularly at first, with caution. One should never cause his heart to work so fast that it cannot handle the increase (from exercising) in the volume of blood or cannot prevent the blood pressure from rising rapidly. It is always bad business to keep on exercising until it takes a long time to recover from fatigue. Walking has the advantage that we can alter the speed and distance traveled to suit our physical condition and stop and rest when necessary.

As Aaron Sussman and Ruth Goode said in their book, *The Magic of Walking*, if our heart rate and blood pressure are high, walking will bring the heart rate and blood pressure to normal.

Man, unlike the four-legged animals, has a circulatory system that works against gravity. In the course of twenty-four hours some 72,000 quarts of blood have been moved over nearly 100,000 miles of "circulatory roads." As we walk, the muscles of the lower and middle parts of our bodies contract and squeeze, forcing the blood along to the heart and brain in spite of gravity.

The old excuse that exercise makes us hungry and increases weight is about the weakest reason one can think of to be lazy. Walkers don't have large waistlines, huge hips, and multiple chins. They are not always complaining about poor elimination, indigestion, and inability to sleep.

Dr. Edward L. Bortz, the great geriatrics researcher, recently said: "We take vigorous exception to the prophets of doom who see only the degeneration of the body with the passing of time. It begins to appear that exercise is the master conditioner for the healthy and the major therapy for the ill."

The best result obtained from physical activity is the development of extra circulatory routes when main coronary arteries are blocked. This building a "second heart" through physical activity worked for generations for our forefathers. When a doctor talks about the danger from stress to a successful businessman, he is talking about the danger to the man's heart resulting from his changed living habits. The man has two or more automobiles so he doesn't walk. He has moved from his two-story home to a fashionable apartment and doesn't climb stairs. He overeats and drinks too much at his club at noon. Since he is an executive, he doesn't walk around the plant any more but sits behind a desk while working. When he gets home, he has to have a few drinks "to relax" and get ready for a big dinner. Is that too much stress, or is it asking for coronary thrombosis?

Drs. Kenneth Cooper and Kevin Brown of the United States Air Force Medical Corps in a new book, *Aerobics*, state that the best exercise for cardiovascular health is that which demands oxygen and compels the body to process and deliver it. *Aerobics* resulted from four years' study of five thousand officers and airmen and the amount of daily and weekly exercise needed to produce and maintain cardiovascular health.

Several heart researchers, Drs. Kenneth Cooper, M. J. Karvonen, Michael Pollack, and others have told us that after a training period to improve cardiovascular fitness the pulse rate is lower when we are resting.

I am not saying that exercise will prevent heart attacks. Exercise, in moderation, is good for the heart, but it is only one step toward heart health. We must also have proper nutrients–vitamins and minerals–and maintain an interest in life.

12 THE BLIND TRY TO LEAD THE BLIND

ABOUT THREE YEARS ago I received a long distance call from a lady on the east coast. She said a friend had given her two of my health books and she hoped I could send her to a physician who might help her. She said her family physician had diagnosed her as a hypochondriac and a neurotic and had sent her to a psychiatrist who had given her tranquilizing drugs and shock treatments. I told her that I knew no doctor in her city, but that I had read some excellent articles in the medical journals written by a psychiatrist of that city. I gave her the name of the physician and told her I could not recommend him as all I knew about him was what I had just told her.

A year later a good-looking young couple walked into my office. She told me that I would never know how much I did for her by giving her the name of a wonderful physician. She said: "The doctor told me I should have a thorough physical examination. When that was done, he said I was suffering from hypoglycemia, or low blood sugar, and that I needed hormones and vitamins. I asked if I would need to take tranquilizers and shock treatments. His answer was, 'Most hypoglycemics cannot tolerate tranquilizing drugs. I have never heard of a low blood sugar sufferer who was helped by tranquilizers. You should never permit another physician to give you shock treatments.' "

She continued: "With this doctor's help, I became a new person. I lost thirty pounds with no effort on my part and I have more pep and vitality than I ever had before. I went back to work a few months ago. For the first time in years I am really alive."

Both the husband and wife seemed worried about whether the shock treatments had injured her brain. I said: "I am no physician, but I don't think you suffered any permanent injuries from the treatments. Shock treatment for mental illness isn't new. The caveman used it; since he didn't have electricity he took a club and tried to knock the one he thought was not normal into his senses." I asked her what would have happened if she hadn't found this psychiatrist who never forgot that he was a physician. She told me she was seriously considering suicide the day she called me. The husband was bitter about the experiences with the first psychiatrist. He remarked: "I think it was a case of the blind trying to lead the blind."

During the past few years I have visited with many men and women who had suffered serious heart attacks. I was anxious to know what each one was doing to avoid future attacks. Apparently, the only dietary instructions given by their doctors were not to eat saturated fats and to take off weight. None of them had been warned of the dangers of eating sugar and I noticed that all of them used salt to season their foods.

About half of those I talked with were taking drugs to lower blood pressure. Nearly all of them were on some kind of prescribed medication to lower the blood cholesterol level.

More than half of those interviewed were taking vitamin supplements "on their own." If their physicians knew that vitamin B_3 (niacin or niacinamide) lowers blood cholesterol, they apparently had not shared that information with their patients.

One lady heart victim told me that she asked her doctor about vitamins. She said he gave her a lecture on the danger of vitamin poisoning and concluded by saying: "If you take a small glass of orange juice each day, you will get all the vitamins and minerals you need." She stated that her daughter, a college freshman who had taken home economics courses in high school, heard what the doctor said and remarked: "That was the most stupid thing I ever heard about vitamins. No wonder he thinks vitamins are poisons."

All heart patients are told to avoid stress. From the information given me, I concluded that none had eaten unsaturated fats excessively before they had heart attacks and all of them were trying to eat polyunsaturated fats. Not one of them admitted having used lard or fat meats. All denied having eaten eggs, butter, cream, or cheese to excess. Nearly all said they were overweight and had not exercised regularly before they became ill.

I am certain that if you take a poll of your friends who had serious heart trouble and ask each one if he or she believes that stress and/or eating animal fats caused their difficulties, you will get more negative than positive answers.

Most doctors believe that heart attacks run in coronary-prone families. Much has been written by researchers on "hereditary" atherosclerosis, hypertension, hypercholesteremia, obesity, hyperlipemia, and diabetes. While this kind of medical literature makes interesting reading, it has no place in a book to show how heart attacks can be prevented as none of us had anything to do with selecting our ancestors. If you, like I, come from a family with a bad coronary history, you must be careful to observe the rules for a healthy heart. I do not feel that I am in any more danger of a cardiovascular disease than if I came from a family free of heart ailments.

A few months back I went through a new high school building in one of our Oklahoma cities. The school cafeteria was completely lined with dispensing machines for sugared soft drinks and candy bars. I was told that all of the other city schools followed this pattern as to drinks and candy. The city was spending millions of dollars for fine buildings, wonderful equipment, excellent teachers, and other proper expenditures. I thought how foolish it was to prepare boys and girls for adult life and at the same time make sugar so available and attractive that diabetes, heart disease, cancer, and a host of other ailments will later overtake many of them.

There is no need of kidding ourselves; we are a nation of medicine-takers and conditions are getting worse instead of better. On every hand we hear the prophets of doom say that America "is falling apart at the seams." If one picks up a daily newspaper and reads what is going on in our courts, on our college campuses, on the streets of our cities, and in some of our churches, he wonders about our national sanity.

Our scientists have successfully discovered remedies

that counteract poisoning by acids, alkaloids, glycosides, metals, snake bites, and dangerous drugs. If some of our men and women of genius can come up with an antidote against sugar poisoning, it will be the discovery of the century!

Dr. Howard Burchell of Mayo Clinic reported in a recent medical journal: "We still have the serious problem of an individual assured by a competent cardiologist that he had a normal heart . . . and yet died that day of an acute myocardial infarction." Heart specialists have told us that postmortem examinations of aged persons who died from heart attacks showed that *three out of four had previous unknown myocardial infarctions.* From these and other medical articles it is a reasonable assumption that a majority of men who reach the age of 65 have one or more heart scars produced by former attacks that were so mild they never knew they had infarctions.

We say that Mr. Smith had a sudden heart attack, which is not true. The blockage in Mr. Smith's coronaries which resulted in the coronary thrombosis had been increasing from year to year. His cardiovascular system was in such condition that stress, usually mild —as a big meal, physical exertion, or an emotional upset—precipitated the heart attack.

Medical statisticians have told us that up to the age of 50 men are seven to one more prone to coronary disease than are women. Even in the 50-to-60 group the ratio is five men to one woman. Physicians have informed us that women have a built-in protection against cardiovascular diseases—the female sex hormones.

After the menopause, or following a hysterectomy, women are less subject to coronary diseases than men because they had many years' protection from such diseases by reason of their sex. By the time a wife reaches the menopause stage, her husband, in all probability, has considerable hardening and some narrowing of the arteries.

Don't be angry with your doctor if he gives you prescriptions for drugs to reduce your blood pressure and inhibit blood cholesterol and says nothing about nutrition. Most patients don't want anyone, including physicians, to change their eating habits. They, like millions of other Americans, believe that drugs will cure any condition.

I have known several men who were warned by their physicians that unless they gave up sugar they would become diabetics. They did not give up the sweets but later were pathetic figures who took insulin and died horrible deaths. I have heard middle-aged and older men say they would die rather than not eat foods they liked and had always eaten.

Nutrition is a subject the layman and not the busy doctor should study. Contrary to popular belief, nutrition is not technical, complicated and difficult to understand. Any individual who would have a healthy body and a healthy mind must know what foods he should eat and what foods he must avoid.

I have often been asked what I consider the principal cause of our high-disease rate in America. My answer is always "ignorance and prejudice." When I read in a text-book used in medical schools that "atherosclerosis is a disease of old age," when I hear doctors testify in court that "senility is inevitable with advanced years," and when I hear doctors condemn taking supplements except "by prescription," I realize how important it is for every layman to have a knowledge of nutrition.

Selig Greenberg in his book, *The Quality of Mercy*, said: "It is adults and not teenagers who are the main consumers of the more than 220 million prescriptions for mood-affecting drugs written annually by physicians, often without regard either for the underlying causes of their patient's distress or the possible addictive and other adverse effects of these compounds. . . . The explosive proliferation of drugs—there are now about 21,000 different drugs in the American marketplace—has led to an overmedicated society—is crowding our hospitals with the one and a half million people every year suffering from adverse reactions to doctor-prescribed drugs.

"Gaudy promotion of this flood of new preparations has so confused the nation's physicians that they are prescribing new medications without sufficient knowledge of their side effects or long-range properties. Beguiling drug advertising has to a substantial degree replaced formal post graduate medical education. Legal controls on the manufacture and distribution of medications are grossly inadequate," reported Greenberg.

Dr. Isabel Jennings in her book, *Vitamins in Endocrine Metabolism*, pointed out the necessity for diabetics to take two other B vitamins, riboflavin and pantothenic acid. She mentioned that the diabetic must take vitamin A supplements because, for some unknown reason, he cannot make use of vegetable sources to produce vitamin A in his body. I doubt if one doctor in a hundred has informed his diabetic patient that he is dependent on supplementation for vitamin A. Dr. Jennings corroborated Dr. Evan V. Shute's contention that vitamin E has been found to reduce insulin requirements of diabetics.

If your father who has lived alone since the death of your mother can't remember what day of the week it is, forgets where he was supposed to meet you downtown, and can't recall where he left things, don't jump at the conclusion he is turning into a vegetable because he is over 70 years old. Give him vitamin and mineral supplements, particularly substantial amounts of vitamins B and C, and the chances are he won't have to be sent to a nursing home or a hospital.

Drs. F. I. Shuman and R. I. Goldberg, Boston physicians, reported in the June 1965 *Journal of the American Geriatrics Society*, spectacular success with aged patients with apparent enfeebled mentalities by feeding them vitamin B_3 (niacin or niacinamide), one 100-mg. tablet with each meal, and a daily multivitamin supplement.

An Oklahoma banker who lived alone following his wife's death went to several physicians with numerous health complaints. He became too ill to continue working and, at the urging of a daughter, went to the Mayo Clinic where he was found to be suffering from scurvy, a vitamin C deficiency disease. When huge amounts of ascorbic acid were given, he quickly regained his health. The fact that he was wealthy and could afford any food he needed was sufficient reason for the Oklahoma doctors to ignore the question of malnutrition.

Every year hundreds of thousands of women in America go on reducing diets that make them more attractive and usually younger looking. They are, unfortunately, not always happier, because they often suffer a myriad of anxiety symptoms—such as fear of heart disease, insanity, and some other unknown but terrible doom. They have heart palpitation, difficulty in breathing, tremors, and weakness.

The physicians from whom they seek help prescribe tranquilizers and suggest psychiatric help. What most of these dieters should have known is that when one reduces his or her food intake, the necessary vitamins and minerals cannot be lowered, much less omitted, without dangerous consequences.

Sometimes these people, after vitamin and mineral therapy, continue to suffer anxiety neurosis. Drs. Ferris Pitts, Jr., and James McClure, Jr., psychiatrists of the Washington University school of medicine, in the December 21, 1967, *New England Journal of Medicine*, presented a scientific study of the cause of anxiety neurosis and what can be done to correct it. Heretofore, when one had unreasonable fears, was jumpy, couldn't keep from shaking, had trouble breathing, and the like, conventional Freudian concepts of childhood neuroses prevailed with psychiatrists.

Drs. Pitts and McClure found that physical exercise made these patients worse, which led them to believe that excess lactic acid was the cause of the anxiety neurosis. Tests proved the correctness of this theory. Since the body produces lactic acid, which is indispensable to life, these psychiatrists set out to find what counteracts the effects of excess lactic acid. They found that calcium would overcome the anxiety symptoms of their patients.

When you have symptoms of choking, smothering, nervous chill, palpitation, tremors, and unreasonable fears, before you start a long and expensive psychotherapy course of treatment and take tranquilizing drugs try these things:

1. Eliminate sugar from your diet.
2. Take an ample amount of calcium, preferably bone meal, and of course you will need vitamin D to help you absorb calcium.
3. If you are more nervous and tense following physical exertion, reduce the amount of exercise until you get the anxiety problem under control. Then you can gradually increase the exercise without any resulting distress from excessive lactic acid.

How calcium deficiency causes one to be overly anxious is not known. An error in glucose metabolism causes the production of too much lactic acid. Probably, calcium combines with lactate around the sensitive nerve endings to overcome the irritations that make us nervous and overly anxious without cause.

Dr. Hans Selye believes that stress is the primary cause of disease and aging. Research conducted at Tulane University school of medicine revealed that stress can activate latent diseases. (*New York Times*, June 11, 1970.)

Our old friend, vitamin E, is first in its ability to help us overcome the effects of stress. As Dr. Selye has so forcefully demonstrated, vitamin E prevents premature aging and reverses the aging process when already begun. Dr. G. A. Goria, an Italian physician, has shown that vitamin E can and does improve the functioning of a normal heart as well as the circulatory processes of the body.

Herbert Bailey, famous science writer, in his book, *Vitamin E, Your Key to a Healthy Heart*, said of vitamin E: "You can hardly name a human purpose that is not aided by large amounts of this vitamin. It is the miracle of modern medicine–unfortunately, still undiscovered by too many."

Vitamin B_{12} helps us to withstand stress. Dr. J. MacDonald Holmes in *Medical News* (April 1967) told us that a deficiency of vitamin B_{12} can bring symptoms of tingling sensations in the limbs, numbness, shooting pains, feelings of too hot or too cold, stiffness and weakness of muscles, blunted sensations of touch, pain, and temperature.

Vitamin B_{12} deficiency results in myelin sheath lesions (destruction of a substance which forms a protective sleeve around nerve fibers). Mental symptoms appear in more than half of those with myelin lesions, which are generally cleared up with adequate vitamin B_{12}.

Vitamin C is important as an antistress food principally because it prevents fatigue. In addition to calcium, we know that magnesium plays a part in our ability to remain relaxed and cool when others around us are suffering anxiety attacks and the breakdown of essential body glands and organs. We cannot avoid stress but nutrition will enable us to withstand it without precipitating a heart attack or some other disease of the circulatory system.

The important thing to remember is that stress is a part of life. When we read that Harry Lewis, well beyond 100 years old, works full time as a San Francisco waiter and runs six miles every day, we can understand the fallacy of those who are always talking about the "diseases of age."

Dr. Heinz Wolterek said in his book, *A New Life in Later Years*, "If there is any secret to staying young longer, or prolonging life, the secret is work. Man must use his organs if he wants to stay healthy and active."

As Dr. E. J. Steiglitz said in his book, *The Second Forty Years*, the mind and the body must be kept going, keeping alive the sense of pride and self-reliance. Those who become a prey to heart disease or suffer from any cardiovascular ailments–whether young, middle-aged, or old–have failed to observe the laws of good health.

We read about the debates in Congress between those who want to use billions of dollars of public funds to provide more hospitals and a greater number of physicians, and those who have other plans for national health, as compulsory insurance.

The major argument is over the means of financing a "disease-care" program for all of the people. Some want the government to foot the entire bill; others contend the government should pay part of the costs and individuals and their employers should pay the remainder.

Is this another case of the blind trying to lead the

blind? Will doubling the number of beds in our hospitals and educating twice as many men and women for the medical profession as are now attending medical schools materially reduce the number of heart attacks occurring each year? The answer is an emphatic "no."

Dr. E. Ginzberg, Columbia University economist, said recently: "Despite the substantial increases in expenditures for medical care, there has been no significant increase in male longevity during the past decade." At least four national studies have shown that annual physical checkups have not decreased mortality rates.

Dr. Victor Fuchs, another famous economist, said that the greatest potential for improving the health of the American people "is to be found in what the people do for themselves."

Sweden has 83 doctors for 100,000 people, but only half the death rate of middle-aged men as in the United States. America has 140 physicians per 100,000 population, and we go to our doctors twice as often as do the Swedes.

The truth of the matter is that the knowledge of nutrition most of us have is from advertising from the food industries which is mostly false and misleading.

We boast of having the best medical care and the finest food supply in the world. The obituary columns in our daily newspapers tell a different story. Men of all ages die of coronary thrombosis in greater numbers every year. Our hospitals are crowded to capacity and our physicians complain of being overworked.

Dr. Robert S. Harris, head of the Nutritional

Biochemical Laboratories of Massachusetts Institute of Technology, after a long-term study recently said: "The humble Indians and Mestizos in Mexico suffer less from malnutrition than does the average middle-class family in the United States."

In the November 20, 1967, issue of *The New York Times* is a report from correspondent Max Frankel of what he found in a trip across the nation to find out the thinking of Americans. The temper of the people was described as "unhappy, unpleasant, unfriendly and dissatisified." He found that the people were "eating well."

No nutritionist can better describe a people who are "eating well," perhaps too well, but are suffering from malnutrition. A human body that is deprived of essential nutrition, no matter how much food is put into it, is not the body of a happy, pleasant, friendly, and satisfied person.

One of the best examples of the blind trying to lead the blind is the frequently made statement by physicians that polyunsaturated fats will reduce the incidence of heart attacks. What is worse is that advertisements in medical journals and in popular magazines have claimed that certain named margarines and oils will prevent heart disease and should be used by persons who have suffered coronary heart disease.

The obvious motive behind such advertising is for certain industries to make greater profits from the sales of specified vegetable fats.

After a thirteen years' attempt by a large number of physicians to show that cholesterol levels were lowered in their patients who ate a polyunsaturated diet, there has been no clinical proof to substantiate such theory. On the contrary, it has been shown by Drs. Kritchevsky and Altschule (*Medical Counterpoint*, March 1969) that heating an unsaturated oil to 220° F. for 15 minutes (far less than normal home cooking time and temperature) enhanced atherosclerosis in animals.

The World Health Organization recently reported that during the past thirteen years these changes occurred:

1. In America there was an increase in mortality from atherosclerotic disease.

2. Heart disease decreased 14 percent in Japan where there had been a tremendous increase since 1955 in the consumption of animal fats, eggs, and dairy products.

Removal of cyclamates from the market was based on inferential animal studies. Why do physicians permit false and misleading advertisements regarding polyunsaturated fats to appear in their professional journals? The evidence of the dangers to man from heated polyunsaturates is far greater than was the proof that cyclamates can be harmful. No action has been taken against those concerns which have attempted to influence both physicians and laymen for financial gain by advertisements claiming that polyunsaturates have therapeutic value in coronary heart disease, although the FDA has threatened to prosecute any manufacturer who promoted polyunsaturates as a preventative of heart disease.

While the controversy over cholesterol and its role in heart disease is far from settled, what we are witnessing is that the medical profession and the FDA have allowed commercialism to take over for private gain and control the thinking of doctors and patients on the role of cholesterol in heart disease.

Dr. Edwin R. Pinckney recently said:

"My newest research, and I have well over 300 references to support my views, shows the severe adverse effects of ingesting too much polyunsaturates. We now eat 5 per cent in our diets; the American Heart Association is proposing an increase to 25 per cent; and we find that 10 per cent or more can cause death in animals—or, if the animal lives, it develops intestinal obstruction from the varnish that comes from excessive polyunsaturates (in one instance, where the varnish did pass through the bowel, the animals were found stuck to their cage-floors by their feces).

"We can show an increase in cancer, aging, and many other diseases, including heart disease, in proportion to an increase in polyunsaturates in the diet. The increase in cancer has now been found in *humans* with *no* increase whatever in preventing heart attacks. . . . There is no scientific evidence to connect cholesterol levels with heart attacks or to connect any diet (other than being overweight) with heart disease. . . .

"But in spite of all evidence to the contrary, the primary emphasis toward the control of heart disease today is still directed toward the dietary use of polyunsaturates to lower a patient's serum cholesterol. . . . When available data is gathered and studied, the only proper conclusion seems to be that there is no real evidence that altering a patient's diet—with the stress on polyunsaturates–will treat existing heart disease or prevent future attacks. In a study of firemen, some of whom had abnormally high serum lipids, it was concluded that substitution of unsaturated fat carried no benefits that could be clinically measured or observed."

(With permission from Edward R. Pinckney, M.D., M.P.H., F.A.C.P.)

The high consumption of sugar in America is far more dangerous to the physical and mental health of our people than is the use of cigarettes. I enthusiastically approve everything that has been done to show the dangers of cigarette smoking and to reduce the sales of cigarettes.

Instead of spending billions of dollars annually to try to prolong the lives of those whose health has been wrecked by too much sugar intake, Congress should put such a high tax on sugar that its consumption is lowered to a fourth of what is now sold each year. As is done with cigarettes, a warning that sugar is dangerous to health should be printed on the container of every package of sugar sold.

When more than one hundred fifty cardiovascular specialists publicly admit that there is no proof that fats and cholesterol cause heart disease in man (report from Inter-Society Commission for Heart Disease Resources, released December 1970), is it not time for American physicians to forget discredited and outworn *theories* of what causes heart attacks and how heart disease can be avoided? What excuse can they offer for being so opposed to trying nutrition as a preventive of cardiovascular diseases?

The heart attack you are statistically scheduled to suffer can be avoided *by you*. The rules to follow for a healthy heart are not complicated or difficult. The happiness that comes from better physical and mental health through good nutrition is greater than can be imagined.

GLOSSARY

ANGINA PECTORIS.

A chest pain, with a feeling of suffocation and impending death, due most often to absence or lack of oxygen of the middle and thickest layer of the heart wall composed of cardiac muscles. Angina pectoris is usually precipitated by effort or excitement.

AORTA.

The main trunk from which the systemic arterial system proceeds. It arises from the left ventricle of the heart.

ARTERIOSCLEROSIS.

A chronic disease characterized by abnormal thickening and hardening of the arterial walls.

ATHEROMA.

Arteriosclerosis with marked degenerative changes.

ATHEROSCLEROSIS.

A lesion of large- and medium-sized arteries with deposits of plaques containing cholesterol, lipoid or fat materials, and calcium.

CAPILLARY.

A small blood vessel of the vascular system.

CARDIAC.

Relating to the heart. Sometimes used as relating to heart disease.

CHOLESTEROL.

A fatlike substance found in animal fats and oils, in bile, blood, brain tissues, nerve fibers, the liver, kidneys, and adrenal glands.

COLLATERAL CIRCULATION.

An interconnecting system of small arteries connecting with the coronary arteries. They are sometimes capable of sufficient expansion to substitute for a blocked artery and avert a heart attack.

CORONARY.

Relating to the heart. Sometimes used as referring to a coronary artery or vein.

CORONARY THROMBOSIS.

Also called a CORONARY OCCLUSION. The blocking of a coronary artery of the heart by a thrombus, or clot of blood formed within a blood vessel.

DEGENERATIVE DISEASES.

A number of diseases that most often show up in middle-aged or older persons.

EMBOLISM.

A sudden obstruction of a blood vessel by an embolus or abnormal particle (as an air bubble) circulating in the blood.

EMPTY CALORIES.

Foods that have only caloric values.

FIBRINOGEN.

A globulin produced in the liver and converted into

fibrin during clotting of the blood. Fibrin is an insoluble white protein.

HEART ATTACK.
A layman's term for any number of abnormal heart conditions, but generally referring to coronary thrombosis, myocardial infarction, or angina pectoris.

HEMOPHILIA.
Hereditary tendency to uncontrollable bleeding.

HEMORRHAGE.
Copious discharge of blood from blood vessels.

HEPARIN.
A substance found in the liver that prolongs the clotting time of blood. Also refers to a medicine used by physicians. It is thought that heparin inhibits blood clots and regulates fatty particles in the blood.

HYDROGENATE.
To combine, treat with, or expose to hydrogen.

HYPERCOAGULABILITY.
High clottability of the blood.

HYPERTENSION.
High blood pressure.

INFARCTION.
An area of damaged or dead tissue or organ resulting from obstruction of the local circulation by a thrombus or embolus.

Intermittent claudication.

Leg pains thought to result from atherosclerosis or clogged arteries.

Ischemia.

Localized tissue anemia due to obstruction of inflow of arterial blood.

Lipids.

Any of the various substances as fats or other compounds that with proteins and carbohydrates constitute the principal structural components of living cells.

Metabolism.

Chemical changes in living cells by which energy is provided for vital processes, and where new material is assimilated to repair the waste.

Myocardial infarction.

An infarction of muscular tissue of the heart. (See infarction.)

Myocardial necrosis.

Death of heart muscular tissue, usually as individual cells, or in small localized area.

Occlusion.

Stopping up, obstructing, or cutting off. (See coronary thrombosis.)

Polyunsaturated fats.

Rich in unsaturated fats.

Saturated fats.

A hard fat that does not flow at room temperature. Animal fat, as butter or white fat of meat, is a combination of saturated fat and liquid unsaturated oils. Most 100 percent saturated fats are artificial products, extremely hard, with more the appearance of a brittle plastic than a food.

SENILITY.
A physical and mental infirmity often seen in the aged.

THROMBUS.
See coronary thrombosis.

UNSATURATED FAT.
Usually refers to a fat derived from a vegetable type of product, as corn, cotton, soybean, safflower, and so on. It remains liquid at normal temperature.

VERTIGO.
A disordered state in which one suffers from dizziness or a confused state of mind.

APPENDIX A

THE FAT-SOLUBLE VITAMINS

VITAMIN A, also known as the anti-infective or antiophthalmic vitamin.

This vitamin is found in most colored vegetables, many fruits, eggs, dairy products, margarines, liver, and fish liver oils.

Vitamin A has these positive functions:

1. Builds resistance to infections, especially of the respiratory tract.
2. Permits formation of visual purple in the eye, counteracting nightblindness and weak eyesight.
3. Promotes healthy skin.
4. Helps maintain a healthy condition of the outer layers of many tissues and organs.
5. Essential for pregnancy and lactation.
6. Promotes growth and vitality.
7. Increases longevity and delays senility.

A deficiency of vitamin A may result in nightblindness, increased susceptibility to infections, dry and scaly skin, lack of appetite and vigor, defective teeth having a thin and weak enamel, retarded growth, intestinal disorders, and general debility. Other organ systems affected by a deficiency of vitamin A are the digestive system, genitourinary system, special senses, and endocrine system.

An increased need for this vitamin occurs during infancy, pregnancy, and lactation.

An excess of vitamin A is stored in the body. Roughly 95 percent of vitamin A reserves are stored in the liver.

VITAMIN D, also called the "sunshine vitamin," and Viosterol and Ergosterol.

This vitamin is found in fish liver oils, fats, eggs, milk, butter, and sunshine.

The positive functions of vitamin D include:

1. Regulates the use of calcium and phosphorus in the body and is therefore necessary for the proper formation of bones and teeth.

2. Essential for preventing rickets in children.

3. Important for growth and development in infancy and childhood.

4. Necessary for growth and vigor of children.

Deficiency of vitamin D results in these conditions:

A. Various skeletar deformities, as bowlegs, knock-knees, enlargement of the ends of the long bones, curvature of the spine, softening of the skull in infants, and delayed closing of the anterior fontanelle.

B. Swelling and beading of the ribs.

C. Retarded growth and lack of vigor.

D. Muscular weakness.

E. Enlarged parathyroid glands.

F. Low serum calcium and low body phosphorus. Calcium and phosphorus retentions small or negative.

G. Tooth decay.

H. Rickets and osteomalacia.

I. Various emotional and mental disturbances.

Vitamin D excesses are stored chiefly in the liver; also in the skin, brain, spleen, and bones.

Hypervitaminosis D may result from an excessive and prolonged intake of this vitamin, some of the symptoms of hypervitaminosis being vomiting, headache, drowsiness, diarrhea, and loss of appetite for food. Occasionally, we find a misguided mother who administers an abnormally high amount of vitamin D to a young child which may result in serious impairment of health from deposits of excessive calcium in the heart, large vessels, renal tubules, and soft tissue.

VITAMIN E, also known as Tocopherol.

This vitamin is found in wheat germ, whole wheat, green leaves, vegetable oils, meat, eggs, whole grain cereals, and margarine.

The positive functions of vitamin E are:

1. Antioxidant, which preserves easily oxidizable vitamins and unsaturated fatty acids in foods, mixtures, or the body.
2. Necessary for normal reproduction and in helping to prevent sterility.
3. Useful in helping prevent muscular dystrophy.
4. Helpful in the treatment of threatened abortion.
5. Prevents calcium deposits in blood vessel walls.
6. Valuable in treatment of heart conditions and cardiovascular diseases generally.
7. Useful in the prevention of some emotional and mental disorders.
8. Necessary for growth and development of children.
9. Successfully used in treating certain skin diseases.
10. Acts as a regulator of the metabolism of the cell nucleus.
11. Maintains normal permeability of capillaries.

Some of the deficiency symptoms of this vitamin are loss of reproductive powers, muscular disorders, fragility of red blood cells, nervousness, and general weakness.

VITAMIN K, also known as Menadione and the blood-clotting vitamin.

This vitamin is found in alfalfa and other green plants, soybean oils, and egg yolks.

The positive functions of vitamin K are:

1. Essential for the production of prothrombin, a substance which aids the blood in clotting.

2. Important to combat hypoprothrombinemia in the newborn.

A deficiency of vitamin K is caused by nutritional deficiencies, faulty intestinal synthesis and poor intestinal absorption, hepatic injury , and massive hemorrhages.

Deficiency symptoms are prolonged blood clotting time and multiple hemorrhages, as in subcutaneous tissue, thymus, bladder, eye, adrenals, testes, kidney, and brain.

THE WATER-SOLUBLE VITAMINS

THIAMINE, also known as vitamin B_1, thiamine chloride, the antineurotic and the antiberiberi vitamin.

This vitamin is found in dried yeast, rice husks, whole wheat, oatmeal, peanuts, pork, milk, and most vegetables.

The positive functions of thiamine are:

1. Essential for normal functioning of nerve tissue.

2. Necessary for good appetite, normal digestion, and gastrointestinal tonus.

3. Needed for proper metabolism of carbohydrates and fats.

4. Promotes growth.

5. Aids muscular and heart development.

6. Valuable in establishing good mental health.

The deficiency symptoms of thiamine are:

A. In children, impaired growth.

B . Mental depression and irritability.

C. Loss of appetite, loss of weight, and various aches and pains.

D. Constipation.

E. Insomnia.

F. Various forms of beriberi in advanced cases.

Thiamine has perhaps more to do with a healthy nervous system than does any other vitamin. Loss of ankle and knee jerk reflexes, neuritis, muscular weakness in the feet, calf, and thigh are usually indicative of thiamine deficiency. When the deficiency of this vitamin is marked, the subject may have mental instability, inability to remember, vague fears and uneasiness, and ideas of persecution.

Thiamine is not stored in the body; therefore, it should be ingested each day for normal functioning.

RIBOFLAVIN, also known as vitamin B_2.

This vitamin is found in liver, kidney, milk, yeast, cheese, and most foods that contain thiamine.

The positive functions of riboflavin are:

1. Improves growth and promotes general health.
2. Essential for healthy eyes, skin, and mouth.
3. Important for respiration in poorly vascularized tissues.

Deficiency symptoms of riboflavin are:

A. Cataracts.

B. Corneal vascularization, cloudiness, and ulceration.

C. Dimness of vision, burning and itching of the eyes, and impairment of vision.

D. Congestion of the sclera.

E. Abnormal pigmentation of the iris.

F. Atrophy of the epidermis, sometimes with scaling.

G. Lesions on lips and at corners of the mouth.

H. Inflammation of tip and margin of the tongue, sometimes with purplish color.

I. "Sharkskin" appearance over the nose.

J. Impairment of wound healing.

K. Degeneration of nervous tissues resulting in incoordination, mental confusion, and loss of muscular strength in the arms and legs.

NIACIN, also known as vitamin B_3, and nicotinic acid. This vitamin is sometimes manufactured as Niacinamide (Nicotinamide). Niacinamide is more generally used by doctors since it minimizes the burning, flushing, and itching of the skin that often occurs with niacin or nicotinic acid.

Liver, lean meat, whole wheat, yeast, green vegetables, and beans are good sources of vitamin B_3.

Some deficiency signs of this vitamin are:

1. Pellagra, the most marked symptom being inflammation of the skin and tongue.
2. Gastrointestinal disturbance.
3. Dysfunction of the nervous system.
4. Mental depression and irritability.
5. Fatigue, headaches, and vague aches and pains.
6. Insomnia and general weakness.
7. Loss of appetite and loss of weight.
8. Neuritis.
9. Nausea, vomiting, and abdominal pains.
10. Burning hands and feet, pain in the calves, numbness, weakness, and difficulty in walking.
11. Diarrhea.
12. Mental symptoms ranging from loss of memory to stupor or mania.
13. Failing vision.
14. Prostration and death in extreme cases.

A dietary deficiency of vitamin B_3 is usually accompanied by deficiencies of other members of the B-complex, particularly thiamine, riboflavin, and pyridoxine.

Vitamin B_3 is especially important for the proper functioning of the nervous system. It promotes growth, maintains normal function of the gastrointestinal tract, is necessary for metabolism of sugar, and helps maintain normal skin conditions.

While not always true, it may generally be said that the functions and deficiency symptoms of all the members of the B-complex vitamin group are somewhat similar.

PYRIDOXINE, also known as vitamin B_6.

This vitamin is found in meat, fish, wheat germ, egg yolk, cantaloupe, cabbage, yeast, and milk.

The positive functions of pyridoxine are:

1. Aids in food assimilation and in protein and fat metabolism.
2. Prevents various nervous and skin disorders.
3. Needed for the utilization of amino acids.

Deficiency symptoms of pyridoxine are loss of appetite, nausea, vomiting, lethargy, and dermatitis about the eyes, in the eyebrows, and at the angles of the mouth.

Mental confusion, numbness of the hands and feet, impairment of vibration and position sense are also deficiency signs.

BIOTIN, one of the newly discovered members of the B-complex family.

This vitamin is found in yeast and is present in at least minute quantities in every living cell.

The positive functions of biotin are:

1. Promotion of growth.
2. Related to metabolism of fats.
3. Essential in the conversion of certain amino acids.

A deficiency of biotin may be caused by improper diet and impaired intestinal synthesis of microorganisms. Researchers have found that raw egg white fed to animals will destroy biotin.

Biotin deficiency symptoms are:

A. Exhaustion and drowsiness.

B. Muscle pains and loss of appetite.

C. A type of anemia complicated by skin disease.

In addition to foods containing biotin, this vitamin is synthesized by intestinal flora.

PANTOTHENIC ACID, also known as calcium pantothenate, another member of the B-complex family.

This vitamin is found in liver, kidney, yeast, wheat, bran, peas, and crude molasses.

The positive functions of pantothenic acid are:

1. Necessary for normal digestive processes.

2. Required for synthesis of antibodies.

3. Helps to build body cells and to maintain normal skin, growth, and development of central nervous system.

Pantothenic acid is essential for all living organisms, including man, and was formerly called "the anti-gray hair vitamin," as it was believed to be a factor in restoring gray hair to its original color. This function of the vitamin has not been substantiated.

Deficiency signs of the vitamin are:

A. Retarded growth.

B. Painful and burning feet.

C. Digestive disturbances.

D. Skin abnormalities.

E. Dizzy spells.

F. Diarrhea with bloody stools.

G. Mental and emotional disturbances—subjects becoming discontented, quarrelsome, irascible, easily upset, and antagonistic.

H. Rapid heart rate on exertion.

I. Epigastric distress and constipation.

J. Numbness and tingling of hands and feet.

K. Weakness of the extensor muscles of the fingers.

This vitamin is related to the utilization of other vitamins, especially riboflavin, and depends also on the availability of folic acid and biotin. It is involved in adrenal function.

FOLIC ACID, another member of the B-complex family.

This vitamin is found in yeast, liver, kidney, and deep green leafy vegetables.

The positive functions of folic acid are:

1. Essential to the formation of red blood cells by its action on the bone marrow.

2. Aids in protein metabolism and contributes to normal growth.

3. Action related to that of ascorbic acid (vitamin C).

Deficiency symptoms of the vitamin are:

A. Nutritional macrocytic anemia.

B. Endocrine disturbance.

VITAMIN B_{12}, also known as the "red vitamin," and a member of the B-complex family.

This vitamin comes from liver, beef, pork, eggs, milk, and cheese. It is also formed by bacterial synthesis.

The positive functions of vitamin B_{12} are:

1. Aids in the formation and regeneration of red blood cells, thus preventing anemia.

2. Promotes growth and increased appetite in children.

3. Acts as a tonic for adults.

4. Improves mental health.

Deficiency of vitamin B_{12} leads to these symptoms:

A. Nutritional and pernicious anemia.

B. Poor appetite and growth failure in childhood.

C. Tiredness.

D. Nervousness, mental confusion, and, in some instances, irrational talk and conduct.

Vitamin B_{12} content is high in the organ meats, as liver, kidney, and so on. It is medium in fish and the muscle meats and low in milk, yeast, soybeans, wheat, and corn.

ASCORBIC ACID, also known as cevitamic acid and vitamin C.

This vitamin is found in citrus fruits, berries, greens, cabbages, and peppers. It is easily destroyed by cooking.

The positive functions of vitamin C are:

1. Necessary for healthy teeth, gums, and bones.
2. Strengthens all connective tissue.
3. Promotes wound healing.
4. Prevents blood clots during and following surgery.
5. Promotes capillary integrity and prevents permeability.
6. Important factor in maintaining sound physical and mental health.
7. May be involved in the absorption and utilization of dietary iron and the maintenance of normal blood hemoglobin levels.
8. Related to the metabolism of certain amino acids.
9. A relationship may exist between vitamin C and the production of adrenal-cortical hormones in view of the high concentration of this vitamin in the adrenals.
10. Blood vitamin A levels are correlated with plasma ascorbic acid contents.
11. Probably a component of a reversible oxidation-reduction system in the body, acting as a hydrogen transporter.
12. Promotes knitting of bones following fractures.
13. Prevents scurvy.
14. Important for healthy skin and eyes.

APPENDIX B

VITAMIN D IN FOODS

(A—micrograms; B—International Units: per 100 g. edible portion)

	A	B
Beef steak	0.33	13
Beet greens	0.004	0.2
Bread, vitamin D	1.7	68
Butter	2.3	92
Cabbage	0.005	0.2
Carrot tops	0.075	3
Cheese	0.83	33
Cod-liver oil	250	10,000
Corn oil	0.22	9
Cream	0.42	17
Crisco	0.22	9
Egg yolk	6.6	265
Halibut-liver oil	3,500	140,000
Herring, canned	8.2	330
Liver, beef, raw	.85	34
Liver, lamb, raw	.45	18
Liver, pork, raw	1.10	44
Liver, veal	0.24	9.6
Mackerel, fresh, raw	27.7	1,100
Milk, whole	0.11	4.4
Milk, vitamin D	1.1	44
Pilchards, canned	18.6	745
Salmon, raw	7.4	297
Salmon, canned	7.8	314
Sardines, canned	34.5	1,380
Shrimp	3.75	150

Spinach	.005	0.2
Tuna	5–8	200–320

VITAMIN E–TOCOPHEROL CONTENT OF FOODS
(Micrograms per 100 g. of fresh material)

	Total	*Tocoph.*
Apples	0.74	0.72
Bacon	0.53	0.44
Bananas	0.40	0.37
Beans, dry navy	3.60	0.10
Beef liver	1.40	1.40
Beef steak	0.63	0.47
Butter	2.40	.....
Carrots	0.45	0.45
Celery	0.48	0.46
Chicken	0.25	0.21
Coconut oil	8.30	3.60
Cornmeal, yellow	1.70	0.84
Corn oil	87	7
Cottonseed oil	90	56
Eggs, whole	2.00	1.16
Grapefruit	0.26	0.25
Haddock	0.39	0.35
Lamb chops	0.77	0.62
Lettuce	0.50	0.29
Margarine	54	28
Oatmeal	2.10	1.94
Onions	0.26	0.21
Oranges	0.24	0.23
Peanut oil	22	11
Peas, green	2.10	0.10
Potatoes, sweet	4.0	4.0
Potatoes, white	0.06	.....
Pork chops	0.71	0.63

Rice, brown	2.40	1.20
Soybean oil	140	10
Tomatoes	0.36	0.27
Turnip greens	2.30	2.24

VITAMIN K–DIETARY SOURCES

(Micrograms per 100 g. of edible portion)

Alfalfa	425–850
Cabbage	250
Cauliflower	275
Carrots	10
Corn	10
Liver, pork	115–230
Mushrooms	7
Oats	75
Peas	7
Potatoes	20
Soybeans	190
Spinach	334
Strawberry	13
Tomato, green	49
Tomato, ripe	24
Wheat	36
Wheat bran	80
Wheat germ	37

PYRIDOXINE (VITAMIN B_6)–DIETARY SOURCES

(Micrograms per 100 g. of edible portion)

Apple	26
Asparagus, cnd.	30
Banana	320

Barley	320–560
Beans, green, cnd.	32
Beef	230–320
Beer	50–60
Beet greens	37
Brains, beef	160
Cabbage	120–290
Cantaloupe	36
Cauliflower	20
Carrot, raw	120–220
Cheese	98
Cod	340
Corn, cnd.	68
Corn, yellow	360–570
Corn grits	200
Cottonseed meal	1,310
Eggs, fresh	22–48
Flounder	100
Grapefruit juice	8–18
Grapefruit sections	17–24
Halibut	110
Heart, beef	200–290
Honey	4–27
Kidney, beef	350–990
Lamb	250–370
Lemon juice	35
Lettuce	71
Liver, beef	600–710
Liver, calves	300
Liver, pork	290–590
Malt extract	540
Milk, whole	54–110
Milk, dry	330–820
Milk, dry skim	550
Molasses, blackstrap	2,000–2,490
Oats, rolled	93–150

Onions	63
Orange juice, cnd.	16–31
Orange juice, fresh	18–56
Peaches, cnd.	16
Peanuts	300
Peas, cnd.	46
Peas, dry	160–330
Pork	330–680
Potato	160–250
Raisins	94
Rice, whole	1,030
Rice, white	340–450
Rye	300–370
Salmon, cnd.	450
Salmon, fresh	590
Sardines, cnd.	280
Soybeans	710–1,200
Spinach, cnd.	60
Strawberries	44
Tomatoes, cnd.	710
Tuna, cnd.	440
Veal	280–410
Watermelon	33
Wheat bran	1,380–1,570
Wheat germ	850–1,600
White flour	380–600
Yams	320
Yeast, bakers'	620–700
Yeast, brewers' dry	4,000–5,700

BIOTIN–DIETARY SOURCES

(Micrograms per 100 g. of edible portion)

Bananas	4
Beans, dried lima	10

Beef	4
Carrots	2
Cauliflower	17
Cheese	2
Chicken	5–10
Chocolate	32
Corn	6
Eggs, whole fresh	25
Filberts	16
Grapefruit	3
Halibut	8
Hazel nuts	14
Liver, beef	100
Milk	5
Molasses	9
Mushrooms	16
Onions, dry	4
Oysters	9
Peas, fresh	2
Peas, dried	18
Peanuts, roasted	39
Pork, bacon	7
Pork, muscle	2–5
Salmon	5
Spinach	2
Strawberries	4
Tomatoes	2
Wheat, whole	5

PANTOTHENIC ACID–DIETARY SOURCES
(Micrograms per 100 g. of edible portion)

Beans, dried lima	830
Beef, brain	2,140–2,860

Beef, heart	2,100–2,470
Beef, kidney	3,400
Beef, liver	5,660–8,180
Beef, muscle	1,100
Bread, whole wheat	570
Bread, white	400
Broccoli	1,400
Cauliflower	920
Cheese	350–960
Chicken	530–900
Eggs	2,700
Lamb	600
Lamb, kidney	4,330
Milk, whole	290
Mushrooms	1,700
Oats	1,300
Oranges	340
Oysters	490
Peas, fresh	600–1,040
Peas, dried	2,800
Peanuts, roasted	2,500
Pork, bacon	280–980
Pork, ham	340–660
Pork, kidney	3,140
Pork, liver	5,880–7,300
Pork, muscle	470–1,500
Potatoes, Irish	400–650
Potatoes, sweet	940
Salmon	660–1,100
Soybeans	1,800
Veal chop	110–260
Wheat, whole	1,300
Wheat, germ	2,000
Wheat, bran	2,400

FOLIC ACID CONTENT OF FOODS
(Micrograms per 100 g. edible portion)

	Total Folic Acid	*Free Folic Acid*
MEAT, EGGS		
Beef		
Round steak	7–17	6.7
Chuck	15.2	....
Hamburger	5.0	3.6
Heart	3.1	....
Kidney	58.4	....
Liver	294	....
Sweetbreads	22.8	....
Lamb		
Stew meat	1.9	.4
Leg	3.3	....
Liver	276	....
Pork		
Liver	221	....
Loin	2.4	.2
Ham, smoked	7.8	.3
Sausage	12.5	.5
Poultry		
Chicken, dark	2.8	....
Chicken, white	3.1	....
Chicken, liver	377	....
Turkey	3–15	4–12
Eggs		
Whole	5.1	....

	Total Folic Acid	*Free Folic Acid*
White	.6	....
Yolk	12.9	....
NUTS		
Almonds	45.7	....
Brazil nuts	4.5	....
Coconuts	27.6	....
Filberts	66.6	....
Peanuts	56.6	....
Pecans	27.0	....
Walnuts	77.0	....
VEGETABLES, FRESH		
Asparagus	89–142	59.6
Beans, lima	10–58	5.6
Beans, lima, dry	103	10.7
Beans, snap	13–56	10.7
Beans, navy, dry	129	11–33
Beans, wax	15–39	....
Beets	13.5	3.3
Broccoli	33.9	8–14
Brussels sprouts	27.1	11.7
Cabbage	6–42	3.1
Carrots	8	3.1
Cauliflower	29.1	8.5
Celery	7.2	2.5
Corn, sweet	9–79	5
Cucumbers	6.7	3.8
Egg plant	5–15	3.8
GREENS		
Beet	20–50	23.8
Chicory	30	4.9
Endive	27–63	....

	Total Folic Acid	*Free Folic Acid*
Escarole	25.8	...
Kale	50.9	31.0
Mustard	17–38	...
Parsley	42.9	...
Spinach	49–115	31–110
Swiss chard	32–64	5
Turnip	83.4	39.1
Watercress	47.6	...
Kohlrabi	10.1	...
Lentils, dry	99	24.5
Lettuce	4–54	2–12
Mushrooms	14–29	20.5
Okra	24.1	...
Onions, green, with tops	12.6	...
Onions, mature	6–14	...
Parsnips	8–37	7.6
Peas	5–35	4–15
Peas, dry split	22	6.2
Peppers, green	4–11	1.5
Potatoes, peeled	4–12	2–3
Potato peels	14.4	6.6
Potatoes, whole	2–135	3.3
Pumpkin	5–10	4.6
Radishes	3–10	2.7
Rutabagas	3–7	3.3
Soybeans, dry	1.92	91.6
Squash, acorn	16.7	10.1
Squash, crookneck	7–16	5
Squash, zucchini	10.8	...
Sweet potatoes	5–19	...
Tomatoes	2–16	4
Turnips	4.3	...

FRUIT	Total Folic Acid	Free Folic Acid
Apples	.5	....
Apricots	3.6	4
Apricots, dried	4.7	1.6
Avocados	6–57	17.6
Bananas	9.6	6.1
BERRIES		
Blackberries	6–18	14.5
Blueberries	7.6	2.7
Cranberries	1.7	.5
Red raspberries	5.1	3.2
Strawberries	5.3	1.6
Cantaloupes	3–8	8.8
Cherries, Bing	6.5	3.0
Dates, dry	24.7	10.0
Figs	6.7	....
Figs, dry	7–14	4.2
Grapefruit	2.7	1.4
Grapes, green	4.5	1.4
Grapes, red	4.9	3.1
Honeydew melon	4.9	4.1
Lemons	7.4	2.4
Limes	4.6	2.6
Oranges	5.1	2.4
Orange juice	4.8	....
Peaches, yellow	2.3	.6
Pears	2.5	.7
Pineapple	.8–6	1.5
Plums, red	.6–3	.7
Plums, yellow	1.2	.3
Prunes, dry	5.4	3.5

	Total Folic Acid	Free Folic Acid
Rhubarb	2.5	.5
Tangerines	7.4	1.3
Watermelon	.6	.3

CEREALS AND OTHER GRAIN PRODUCTS

	Total Folic Acid	Free Folic Acid
Breads		
Cracked wheat	27	....
Rye	19.8	....
Vienna	11.2	....
White	15	....
Breakfast Cereals		
Cornflakes	5.5	2.8
Cornmeal	6.5	2.4
Corn and soya	80.1	14.2
Oats, ready to eat	22.5	6.3
Oatmeal	30.5	7.8
Wheat bran	100	24–47
Wheat farina	13.6	6.2
Wheat, shredded	29–87	8–28
Flour		
Cake	6.6	....
Rye	18.0	....
White, enriched	8.1	....
Whole wheat	38	....
Grains		
Barley	50	21.0
Corn, yellow	23.6	5.0
Oats, white	23–66	13–26
Rice, brown	22	10.9
Rye	34.4	13.8

	Total Folic Acid	*Free Folic Acid*
Wheat	27–51	.8–30

MILK AND CHEESE

Milk		
Buttermilk	11.1	....
Evaporated milk	.7	....
Cheese		
Cheddar	15.5	....
Cottage	21–46	....
Processed	11.1	....

The foregoing tables reproduced from *Nutritional Data*, 5th Ed. 2nd Rev. printing (1964), with permission of H. J. Heinz Company.